FoodSmart

Understanding Nutrition
In The 21st Century

by Diana Hunter

Consumer Press
Fort Lauderdale, Florida

FoodSmart

Understanding Nutrition
In The 21st Century

Published by:
Consumer Press
13326 Southwest 28th Street, Suite 102
Fort Lauderdale, FL 33330-1102

The author, publisher, and any and all affiliated parties with regard to the production of this book shall have neither liability nor responsibility to any person, property, entity, or organization whatsoever with respect to any loss or damage whatsoever caused, or alleged to be caused, directly or indirectly, by the information contained herein. This book is sold with the understanding that the publisher is not engaged in rendering nutritional, medical, or other professional service. If medical advice or other expert assistance is required, the services of an appropriate professional should be sought. Although all efforts have been made to ensure correctness, the author and publisher assume no responsibility for errors, omissions, or inaccuracies.

Common sense is a virtue. If you are clinically obese, have any other form of health problem, are on medication of any kind, have a family history of any type of disease, or are pregnant or attempting to become pregnant, be sure to consult fully with one or more qualified medical professionals before making nutrition-related lifestyle changes. Good health is a team effort that begins with, and is directed by, you. Even if you believe yourself to be in good or relatively good health, having a qualified medical professional monitor your progress can be an asset. In addition, due to the ever-changing and debatable nature of nutrition, information contained in this book may not reflect every up-to-the-minute perspective.

Library of Congress Cataloging-in-Publication Data
Hunter, Diana, 1961-
Foodsmart: understanding nutrition in the 21st century / by Diana Hunter.
p. cm.
Includes index.
ISBN 978-1-891264-42-9 (pbk. : alk. paper)
1. Nutrition. 2. Health. I. Title.
RA784.H796 2009
613.2--dc22
2009022839

ISBN-10: 1-891264-42-7 $21.95 Softcover
ISBN-13: 978-1-891264-42-9

10 9 8 7 6 5 4 3 2
Printed in the United States of America

Table of Contents

About The Author

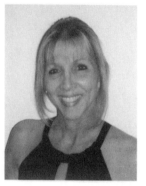

Diana Hunter is an award-winning author and nutritional researcher with dual honors degrees in conventional and holistic nutrition. Her background includes studies and awards in behavioral science.

Ms. Hunter's passion lies in learning about food and nutrients and their effects on the body. This passion began nearly twenty-five years ago after personal health issues involving food prompted her to investigate her diet, and continued to grow as she began researching a multitude of nutritional angles related to motherhood and child development while raising her family. This in turn prompted her to author her previous title, The Ritalin-Free Child: *Managing Hyperactivity & Attention Deficits Without Drugs,* a Parent's Choice Approved book designed to help those who are unable to take medication for hyperactivity and inattention.

Today Ms. Hunter's goal is to help educate others about nutrition and health on a global scale, with a focus on helping those with cancer and other debilitating illnesses.

She is an avid gardener of organic and heirloom fruits, vegetables, and herbs, which she enjoys sharing with family and friends.

She resides in Fort Lauderdale, Florida.

For Brenden and Tony

In loving memory of

Lillian Bessie Pappas and *Anna Lysy*,

who lit a candle that will never burn out.

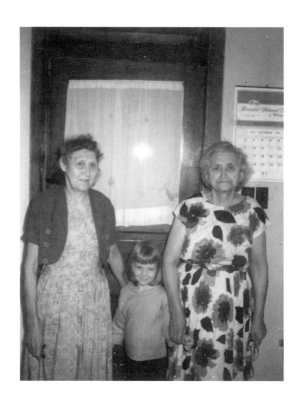

Acknowledgements

Special thanks to my family (Steve, Tony, Brenden, and Cori), Joseph Pappas, Cici Petersen, Kim Nichols, Diane & Vito Lentini, Gerda Williams, Linda Muzzarelli, Gina Muzzarelli, Sam Concialdi, Winona Golden, T. Kim Chesher, Amber Thompson, Shawna Thompson, Lois Norfolk, John Norfolk, Billy Byrne, Laura Precedo-Choudry, Ph.D., Gordon Maddison, Thomas Moeschl, John Collins, Ph.D., Mitchell Samuels, D.O., Charles Shofnos, D.D.S., Arturo Reyna, and the late Betsy Rogers and Jan Nathan.

Special thanks is also extended to the many researchers and others around the globe who provided assistance and permissions during the development of this book, and to Southern WebWorks for their outstanding service and constant willingness to provide the solutions we need at a moment's notice.

Preface

The idea for this book was inspired by the vast and growing need for clarity about nutrition. More of us than ever are in search of clear, definitive answers about what to consume for optimal health. This is due in part to the fact that escalating healthcare costs and high disease rates have led to a full-blown movement of preventive care in which nutrition is at the forefront. As we have come to the realization that what we consume has a major impact on our overall well-being, and that it is an area over which we have much control, our quest for information has intensified. Our interest has also been driven by the increasing awareness that while learning about nutrition requires some effort, it is effort well spent.

Although by nature nutrition is not a perfectly definitive science, we can still develop a solid understanding of the factors that affect it and how to work with them to make the best nutritional choices. The key is to become familiar with the aspects that cause confusion and then effectively redirect them into solutions that enhance our personal health. This book strives to help us achieve that goal as easily as possible. It is designed as both a guide and a reference with the intention of making nutrition a more graspable, useful part of our lives.

Chapters one and two are conceptual. Chapter one takes an in-depth look at many of the situations that lead to misunderstanding about what to consume. Chapter two focuses on the individual considerations that are associated with specific foods, beverages, and other consumables and how we can gather the most accurate information about them. Together these chapters provide a system through which we can finally make sense of nutrition. By learning what causes the confusion, we become less confused, and by knowing how to obtain valid information on nutritional topics and use it to our benefit, we gain a higher degree of control over both our diet and our health.

The remaining chapters concentrate more directly on the known or potential problems and benefits associated with foods, food components, additives, and nutrients, and address other nutrition-related concerns.

Introduction

The world of nutrition is vast and exciting, yet it can also be confusing. While within the last few decades alone much has been brought to light on the nutritional scene, many new and controversial doors have also been opened. Today, issues concerning genetic modification, organics, fat replacements, and other food-related topics regularly make the news. Unfortunately, the information presented is often the opposite of current public knowledge or understanding—a situation that often causes confusion and frustration. This scenario is especially prevalent after products that have been on the market for a number of years are retested, or are subjected to new types of testing. There are, however, several valid reasons for these contrasts in information. Some are scientific, others are not. Most are due to new findings through the use of current technology. A host of factors, from agricultural changes and the effects of nature to variations in experiments and their interpretation, lie behind the mixed messages we receive regarding nutrition. With each finding there exists the potential for additional viewpoints and media attention, creating a never-ending cycle. This is compounded by the fact that there is much left to discover.

Overall, many facets of how nutrition is viewed and interpreted have been affected over the years. As food technology has forged ahead at a stunning pace, the new questions of tomorrow and the unanswered questions of yesterday have come together to create the need for a different comprehension of not only individual aspects of nutrition, but more importantly of how to effectively navigate the nutritional landscape as a whole. This is not as difficult as it may seem. As consumers we can benefit most by being proactive and knowing how to best become educated about nutrition as it affects us individually. In short, learning *how* to learn about nutrition is the key. By utilizing a number of reliable resources and taking an active interest in nutrition, we can gain informed perspectives and make confident nutritional choices.

This book was developed with the consumer in mind. It was written to provide a base point from which we can easily and effectively begin to acquire an accurate awareness about nutrition and attain useful insights into healthful living. It is intended to be a source of little-known facts and answers to frequently asked questions as well as a resource of resources, bringing together the knowledge and findings of numerous researchers to assist us in gaining an edge in maintaining or improving our health. The goal behind it is to help provide clarity about the many aspects of food and to bring to the table an understanding of nutritional research as we progress into the future.

Diana Hunter
June 2009

Chapter 1

$\mathcal{N}$utrition involves a lot of information. It's also constantly affected by change. New foods, products, and technologies are continually being introduced into the foodstream, and differing reports on what's good or bad for us never stop emerging. One day a food, additive, or supplement is beneficial or harmless; the next it promotes cancer, causes us to be overweight, or has some other negative effect. Or vice-versa. Years later the information changes again. For the most part, these fluctuations carry the blame when making sense of nutrition becomes difficult. The actual source of the confusion, however, lies in one factor that answers the question: What causes the information to keep changing? That factor is variables.

In nutrition, variables include every food, nutrient, ingredient, and product as well as the methods by which they are developed, their individual qualities, and the many monetary and health-related scenarios associated with each one. Numerous and unceasing, they affect all aspects of nutritional science and are the reason why research findings on nutrition are often considered to be more a source of frustration than information. These culprits of change exist from the media to the market and beyond, and are responsible for the general lack of definitive scientific answers regarding what we should eat, drink, and take to stay healthy.

Because nutrition is a vast, rapidly growing, and at times imperfect science that is frequently influenced by political and economic factors, it is subject to a high degree of variable activity. The outcomes of this activity often have widespread impact. Consider, for example, the universal effects when the results of a new scientific study on a specific food or additive do not match or even remotely agree with previous research. Since science is continually susceptible to updates in technology, new methods of testing, and differences in viewpoint, it is a major portal through which contradictory information of this nature begins its journey into the public eye. Added to this is the fact that the amount of variables, research studies, and information sources is so overwhelming, the overload alone leads to confusion.

A precise example of variables in action involves the artificial sweetener saccharin, an additive whose history is tantamount to a game of regulatory ping-pong. A synthetic compound derived from coal tar, petroleum, and other sources, this widely used sugar replacement has been repeatedly investigated and reviewed for its potential role in cancer, often with differing results. Scientists, congress, and even presidents have ridden the saccharin merry-go-round, with on-again, off-again proposals suggesting that its use be limited or banned. Discovered by a student researcher at Johns Hopkins University in 1879, it has attracted both national and international scrutiny throughout the years.[1] Its safety still lurks questionably in many minds more than a century later.

The case involving saccharin is only one among numerous instances in which variable activity has left a trail of uncertainty and change. In *Food, Consumers, and the Food Industry* (CRC Press, 2001), Gordon Fuller provides some additional examples in the form of nutrition-related claims and rebuttals that have appeared in popular media over the years: [2]

- Foods with high cholesterol have been bad and good by turns when exogenous cholesterol was found to be not as guilty as suspected in heart disease. Eggs, one common food, were bad, but then became a good source of nutrition in moderation.
- Coffee and chocolate have had checkered histories. Coffee was a cause of pancreatic cancer, but then became a valued nutraceutical. Today, it is a cause of arthritis. Chocolate, a food prone to make its eaters tired, violent, suicidal, depressed, and suffer from migraines, now has health-giving properties and may even be an aphrodisiac.

---

[1] "Regulatory History of Saccharin," *Saccharin,* December 16, 2002, <http://enhs.umn.edu/saccharin/reghistory.html> (March 31, 2006).
[2] Reprinted, adapted, and edited with permission from CRC Press, LLC and Gordon W. Fuller. Copyright © CRC Press, Boca Raton, Florida.

- Butter, an animal source of fat, was condemned as a dietary fat; margarine was good. Now consumers are told that the short-chain fatty acids in butter are good and the trans-acids in margarine are bad. As a result, manufacturing processes have been changed to remove or lower the content of trans-acids in some margarines. Consumers are now not sure what to believe.
- At one time unsaturated fatty acids were very desirable in the diet. Then too much unsaturated fat in the diet was found to be bad for one's heart.
- Saturated fats, specifically those of plant origin, were once condemned as being as bad as animal fats in the diet. They now have been shown to be harmless.
- Red wine in moderation with a meal was once claimed to reduce blood cholesterol, but this finding was challenged—it was the ambience of the meal that contributed to the lowering effect. Then a study found that resveratrol in red wine offsets some of the ill effects of smoking.
- Fiber was a protective factor in preventing colorectal cancers. Then an epidemiological study suggested it did not have any protective action (Fuchs et al., 1999),[3] or if it did it might be due to a genetic link.
- Oats with their fiber were lauded as a potent factor in lowering blood cholesterol. Then they were not. Then another report indicated that a diet rich in oats not only lowers blood cholesterol but regulates blood sugar and lowers blood pressure.
- Beta-carotene, and hence foods high in it, helped prevent cancer of the lung, but then they did not.

These situations and others like them effectively illustrate how variable activity can affect our understanding of nutrition. A major aspect behind the confusion they cause is the fact that they involve several different *types* of nutrition-related variables. Many of these variables involve nature and its wide range of effects on foods, beverages, and other consumables. The rest are related mainly to production, consumption, and experimentation. As

---

[3] Fuchs, C.S., Giovannucci, E.L., Colditz, G.A., Hunter, D.J., Stampfer, M.J., Rosner, B., Speizer, F.E., and Willett, W.C., "Dietary fiber and the risk of colorectal cancer and adenoma in women," *New England Journal of Medicine*, 340, 169, 1999.

each type branches out and combines with the others, our nutritional considerations increase, often becoming more technical as they grow. In general, the greater the number of variables involved and the more diverse they are, the greater the likelihood of confusion. We can get a more concise picture of the kinds of variables that exist by considering them in groups.

The Five Basic Variable Types

There are five primary types of variables that have an influence on nutrition and the industries that surround it:

• Naturally Occurring Variables
• Choice-Related Variables
• Error-Related Variables
• Unknown Variables
• Experimental Variables

Each of these five basic types can exist simultaneously with one or more of the others, to the point where all five occur together. Here we look at each type individually.

1. Naturally Occurring Variables

Naturally occurring variables are those that occur regardless of human intervention, direct or otherwise. The developmental and physical characteristics of foods account for many of them. They include the size, color, and species of consumable plants and animals and the amount of sun and rain food plants receive during growth. They also include the presence or absence of harmful or beneficial insects, many of which have significant widespread effects on food production. Wild honeybees, for example, not only produce honey and pollinate wild-growing and home-grown food plants, but also naturally pollinate large-scale agricultural crops and even provide us with the convenience of seedless watermelons.[4] (The assistance of bees in general in the growth of fruits and vegetables is a major factor in the maintenance of our global food supply.)

Both plants and animals are directly impacted by many of the same nature-induced variables. Whether commercially developed or in the wild, they are each at risk of contracting diseases and encountering other problems due to storms, weather extremes, predators, and changes in the earth's systems of agriculture and aquaculture. Alternately, they can each benefit from a moderate climate, nutrient-filled soil, and a lack of drought. These and other situations often create a domino effect that either improves or impedes on the costs, quality, and availability of plant- and animal-based foods.

The Human Body

Our bodies are also a source of naturally occurring variables that involve nutrition. The rate at which we digest, the amount of nutrients we absorb from the foods we eat, how stress affects our appetite, and how rapidly we lose or gain weight are just a few examples of bodily occurrences that are prone to fluctuation. While we can attempt to control any of these by choice, and often do so successfully, our bodies' natural responses still occur on their own. We simply guide them.

Other considerations include our digestive, dental, and overall states of health, the amount of physical activity we engage in, and our heredity. Each of these factors has an influence on, and is influenced by, nutrition and nature-driven variables. Heredity in particular can biologically predispose us to allergies, cancer, and other conditions including a variety of nutrition-related ailments, though in many instances these are the response to poor diet and unsupported health rather than genetics. Heredity can also provide us with traits that are beneficial, such as the ability to maintain consistently good cholesterol levels regardless of what we eat, though such situations are much less common. (Note that being physically active, avoiding tobacco and

---

[4] Maynard, Donald N. "Growing Seedless Watermelon," *EDIS HS687*, University of Florida IFAS, May 2003, <http://edis.ifas.ufl.edu/CV006> (March 22, 2006).

alcohol, maintaining low stress levels, and regularly consuming cholesterol-*lowering* foods in addition to those that boost cholesterol can also be contributing factors in the ability to maintain good cholesterol levels—and may be learned habits, rather than genetic traits, that have been passed down by previous generations.)

In some cases, race and other hereditary considerations can cause nutrition-related blood test results to be slightly higher than what is considered to be within normal range even though we are otherwise healthy. In these rarer instances the blood levels may be naturally different. Overall, the variables associated with heredity account for part of the reason why a one-size-fits-all approach to nutrition doesn't work.

2. Choice-Related Variables

Nutritional choices generally originate from two or more sources. We usually choose what to consume, while others control how each food or related product is grown or made, where it comes from, or both. For example, farmers, ranchers, and manufacturers make choices related to food growth and production, such as those regarding the use of pesticides, herbicides, fertilizers, and genetic modification, while government agencies decide on regulatory issues, which include setting limits on the types and amounts of chemicals allowed to be used in food development. These situations apply to both domestic and imported foods. However, as other countries often use different processes and are regulated differently, additional variable considerations sometimes arise where imports are concerned. In many instances, packaged foods and beverages are developed utilizing multiple suppliers and ingredients from several countries, with many choices being made by others for better or worse. These situations are obviously lessened in cases where we grow or raise our own foods, or obtain them from known and trusted sources.

Foods

The most obvious and abundant choice-related variables involve the combinations, amounts, and types of foods we consume. Whether to eat them raw or cooked, fresh or canned, or grown by organic or conventional means are only a few considerations in the stream of possibilities. We have options of plant or animal foods derived from land or sea, either locally obtained or imported, and prepared in any number of domestic or cultural ways. We can select specific varieties, how to prepare them, and when to eat them. We can choose them based on fiber, fat, sugar, protein, carbohydrate, or nutrient content. We can also choose them according to brand, price, or ease of preparation. Our options even extend to selecting between irradiated and non-irradiated foods, and those that have or have not been genetically modified. Whether our considerations are based on health, taste, convenience, or any combination of these factors, we are faced with a multitude of selections that affect our health and have a direct bearing on pleasurable, nutritious eating.

Beverages

Water, soft drinks, coffee, tea, alcoholic beverages, juices, milk, and specialty nutritional drinks are among our many beverage choices. We can choose from those developed organically or conventionally and those made from non-irradiated, irradiated, or genetically modified foods. They may be domestic or imported, served hot, cold, iced, or frozen, and may or may not contain additives. We can also choose among those with little or no nutritional value or those packed with nutrients. There are drinks made from plants, animal milks, fruits, and vegetables as well as various types of water-based beverages, all of which may be combined with chemical additives.

Other Choice Factors

We generally make more nutrition-related choices than we realize. Among them are those associated with:

• Supplements
• Diets

- Packaging and storage containers
- Cookware, tableware, and utensils
- Convenience factors
- Personal, psychological, and sociological aspects of nutrition
- Nutritional information sources

3. Error-Related Variables

Errors related to nutrition usually occur during lab research, food production, consumption, or the transfer of information. In the lab, they are represented by miscalculations and mistakes in documentation. In some instances they occur because residues from cleaning products or previous experiments are left inside of supplies and carried over into other experiments. Defective materials and equipment, improper protocol, and tainted or misused chemical substances can also cause errors and lead to distorted research, resulting in large-scale problems. For example, when inaccurate food or supplement analysis occurs, it can lead to the misrepresentation of the quality, nutritive value, or safety of a food or product that affects millions of people. Occurrences like this can hinder nutrition and our understanding of it, and in many cases have the potential to cause serious health effects.

Errors related to food processing and production often involve mechanical failures and the results of improper sanitation. Equipment malfunctions and contamination with bacteria or chemicals can readily disrupt the development and integrity of foods and related products, leading to situations that affect consumption. Some errors are caused when outdated or incorrect ingredients are used in product development or when packaging is filled with a product other than what the label indicates. These situations can occur both in industrial settings and at home, potentially causing reactions, severe illness, or even death.

Other errors related to food processing and production occur while animals are being raised for consumption. For example, the use of contaminated or disease-infested feed can seriously affect livestock, and subsequently the food supply, as witnessed when meat and bone meal from scrapie-infected sheep was fed to cows. The result was Bovine Spongiform Encephalopathy (BSE), also known as Mad Cow Disease.[5] After animals are slaughtered, bullets, needles, and other items are sometimes found in their bodies, accounting for still other errors.

Product labeling is yet another area of production prone to error-related variables. Labels can contain information ranging from accurate to totally unreliable. Failure to list ingredients, improper representation, incorrect naming of ingredients, and inaccurate weights and nutritional values are among the most common problems. Labels can also be torn, illegible, or misprinted. In some instances, specifically those that involve misrepresentation, the errors are intentional; in others they are unintended or due to mechanical errors.

In cases of accidental ingestion, the error-related variables involved may be foods and medications that are incompatible, foods or additives we are allergic or sensitive to, poisonous foods, or contaminated foods. Each can cause negative reactions ranging from mild to life-threatening. There are dozens of food and medication interactions, thousands of potential food allergens, and a number of poisonous foods and food components including certain types of fish, some species of mushrooms, apple seeds, the pits from cherries, and the seeds from within the pits of apricots, peaches, plums, and nectarines.[6] Contaminated foods include those that contain E. coli, Listeria, Salmonella, or other infectious pathogens.

Informational errors made by writers or journalists, or that otherwise occur via the media, are also included in this category. Biased but unfounded viewpoints, distorted perspectives, incomplete facts, and the use of technical language during presentations to mainstream audiences can cause incorrect or misinterpreted information to be released to the public. One missing, incorrect, or elaborate word, a single grammatical error, or a lone case of emphasis

---

[5] United States Food and Drug Administration, Center For Food Safety and Applied Nutrition, September 2005, <http://www.cfsan.fda.gov/~comm/bsefaq.html> (March 27, 2006).

[6] Center For Disease Control. Agency For Toxic Substances and Disease Registry. "ToxFAQs™ for Cyanide." September 2004, < http://www.atsdr.cdc.gov/tfacts8.html> (March 26, 2006).

in the wrong place can easily distort a message. Each of these occurrences can lead to confusion about nutrition and result in negative effects on health.

4. Unknown Variables

Unknown variables exist in four forms:

1) those that are not readily obvious although we know they exist; for example, when we have no idea what types of pesticides, if any, were used on vegetables we are buying at a store or eating in a restaurant;

2) those that we do not have specific knowledge about although we know they exist; for instance, knowing there are B vitamins in a multivitamin without knowing the benefits of B vitamins;

3) those that we do not know exist; and

4) those that have yet to be discovered, such as in cases where a food or nutrient directly appears to be beneficial in some way even though we are uncertain as to the exact mechanism or mechanisms by which it works.

Among the variables that have not been discovered are those that develop when chemical additives are combined, exposed to temperature extremes, or both. These situations are common among gums, candies, snacks, and packaged foods, and in instances where chemical-laden frozen foods are later grilled, baked, fried, or otherwise prepared under heat. In the majority of cases, reactivity between the chemical additives in these products has not been tested. Even with testing we may be unable to secure verified answers as to the exact reactions between such match-ups. Unidentified by-products released due to interactions between chemicals in food products and chemicals added to packaging materials present additional considerations.

In some cases, a product's ingredients vary depending on how, when, or where it is dispensed. We may be unaware of these behind-the-scenes variable differences. For example, it is not widely known that diet sodas purchased in cans or bottles often have different ingredients than the same types sold on tap at restaurants or movie theaters. It is also a less-known fact that coloring may be added to butter, especially during winter months, when most cows have little or no pasture to feed on and therefore intake less beta-carotene from which butter usually gets its yellow tint. In instances like these, variables are often undisclosed on product packaging due to a lack of regulatory requirement. In others they are intentionally kept unknown. According to the U.S. Food & Drug Administration (FDA), companies are permitted to file for exemption from nutrition labeling requirements if the person claiming the exemption employs fewer than an average of 100 full-time employees and fewer than 100,000 units of the product are sold in the U.S. annually. Retailers with annual gross sales of not more than $500,000, or with annual gross sales of foods or dietary supplements to consumers of not more than $50,000 can also request this exemption (see chapter twelve, *Ingredients & Labeling*, for further information). Some companies choose to keep recipes from being duplicated by competitors or others by deeming them "proprietary." Not only are the variables unknown in these situations, but their potential health effects are as well. This is an important consideration when medication interactions, allergies, or sensitivities are a concern.

5. Experimental Variables

Lab experimentation involves a considerable amount of variable activity. Methods of testing, test subjects, supplies, equipment, chemical substances, and temperature all vary, as do the interpretations of experimental outcomes. Both individually and collectively these variables play an integral part in the scientific process from which conclusions about foods, nutrients, and additives are drawn. The slightest variable deviations during the replication of experiments can cause conflicting results. In order for research to be duplicated accurately —a critical facet in proving any theory—every factor involved must either be identical or fall within certain allowable limits proven to the best of our knowledge and ability not to impede on experimental results.

When nutrition-related experiments are performed, their purpose is usually to investigate food safety issues or the relationships between nutrition and a host of other topics including disease, weight control, exercise, sports, brain function, or overall metabolism. This type of research is a foremost source from which we as consumers seek reliable information about what we should consume. Food manufacturers, the FDA, and others, on the other hand, use it to make decisions about the safety and allowable use of foods, beverages, additives, and other consumables. Obtaining such information in a complete, definitive form is difficult due to the fact that each experimental aspect intersects with others on various levels. Not only does this situation result in an influx of *informative* reports that tell us the different effects of foods, additives, and the like, but also in many instances an array of *opposing* reports that disagree about those same effects. It is also the reason why it's not uncommon for a food, food derivative, beverage, herb, or additive to be reported as having benefits as well as negative aspects, or to be deemed as both a cause and a cure. Caffeine is an excellent example, as it is known not only to cause headaches but also to aid in relieving them.

Experimental Animals

A number of different animals, including rodents, rabbits, and pigs, are used in nutritional research. Mice and rats are among the most common and preferred choices. Mice in particular are frequently used due to the fact that, like rats, their genetic makeup closely resembles that of humans.[7] They are also available in many strains (versions of either healthy mice or those that have been genetically altered with differences in everything from immune status to lifespan) and reproduction is generally inexpensive. Their use, however, has limitations. Subtle differences between their genetic patterns and those of humans may have more of an impact than we realize.

---

[7] "The Mouse in Science: Why Mice?" Univ. of Calif. Center for Animal Alternatives, 1996, <http://www.vetmed.ucdavis.edu/Animal_Alternatives/whymice.htm> (March 31, 2006).

Also, mice can't tell us if they are nauseated, have a headache, or have other symptoms that are not obvious through blood tests and standard observation. The overall variable considerations related to experimental animals include species, age, genetics, gender, weight, lifespan, and the number of animals being studied.

While the scientific testing methods that are used to learn how foods and additives affect our bodies often include either animal or human subjects, efficient testing systems and devices are now available that don't require the participation of either one. These include computer models and the use of artificial stomachs in lab settings. In many cases such technology dramatically lessens the need for animal testing or significantly reduces the number of animals used.

Dosage in Animal Testing
The amounts and potencies of substances used in testing are also variable, often differing widely between experiments. Many times excessively large or potent doses are administered to laboratory animals during research that involves drugs, nutrients, or chemical additives. While the purpose of this is to mimic the effects of chronic use and establish safe exposure levels in humans, it can actually create problems or benefits that may never be experienced during minimal or moderate human use.

Human Studies
We do not participate in many types of human experimentation for ethical and practical reasons; more often our roles are confined to taking part in studies or other forms of research that are non-invasive or minimally invasive with little risk. Race, gender, age, weight, and health status are common variables in these cases. When blood, saliva, or other bodily fluids are used to analyze how foods, nutrients, or additives affect the body, however, they too become experimental variables. Blood varies by type, may have more or less clotting ability, and can harbor disease, while the pH of saliva varies not only in the body but from person to person. Genetic differences are also of

growing importance and are likely to play major roles in nutritional research in the future.

Placebos

Placebos exist in the form of pills, injections, therapies, and surgeries. They are often administered to a percentage of the participants in experimental trials to help determine the effects of actual substances or methods of cure. There is some question as to the inertness of those that contain sugar, artificial colors, or drugs, however, as each of these can cause various reactions when taken in extremely minute amounts. As renowned researcher Beatrice Golomb, M.D., Ph.D. has noted, in actuality no substances are known to be physiologically inert; also, no regulations govern what goes into placebos and their components are generally not disclosed.[8] In addition, Dr. Golomb notes that when companies design and manufacture their own placebos, there is the risk that each placebo may be steered further from being inert. All active substances used to produce placebos are considered to be experimental variables.

Other Considerations About Variables & Research

In addition to their other effects on research, variables also cause confusion by making science appear ineffective and unreliable. The influence they have on our ability to develop conclusive scientific evidence about nutrition is not only constant, but considerable. While there is much we have learned, in actuality the overall health risks and benefits of most if not all foods and nutrition-related products are still unknown. This is because science performed to the best of our ability, utilizing the most technological means of research, cannot and does not encompass every possible variable. Consider the use of identical twins in medical and nutritional studies. While the purpose of such

---

[8] Golomb, B.A., "Paradox of Placebo Effect," *Nature,* 1995; 375:530. Reprinted by permission from Macmillan Publishers Ltd.

experimentation has been to explore the effects of specific foods, products, and dietary variations in humans who are genetically equivalent (an ideal testing scenario), in truth we have never been certain that each such twin is actually identical at every level. In fact, studies have now shown that they have some distinct biological differences.[9] Despite our advances, unknown variables still exist in this area of science at genetic and molecular levels we have yet to uncover. We can only see as far as technology and reason will allow us to look. Therefore we inherently make assumptions in the realm of good science.

Good, Debatable Science

Further impeding on our quest to secure concrete answers about nutrition is the fact that theories are disputable. Science and deliberation go hand in hand. The best of what science has to offer has been evaluated from every known angle, rigorously tested, and heavily reviewed. It is not uncommon for tests and reviews to be performed on a food or substance years, decades, or even a century or more after its initial assessment, as in the case of saccharin. Even the most scrutinized research with a narrowed focus may be debated by other scientists or researchers at any time. Variables are the reason. While substantial proof may exist to back a theory, new findings can still surface and viewpoints can still fluctuate.

While some aspects of nutritional science are viewed as more or less definitive, they too are open to review. The process can prove to be beneficial. New technologies often allow us access to answers that help fill in the blanks in previous theories. They also provide us with the opportunity to discover additional information about foods and substances and how they affect our bodies. While this can undoubtedly lead to further investigation of nutritional issues within the scientific community, it is also a step forward in developing the fullest understanding of what to include and avoid in our diets in order to maintain the best state of health.

---

[9] Wagner, Holly, "Identical Twins May Have More Differences Than Meets The Eye," *Ohio State University, Research News*, July 2005, <http://researchnews.osu.edu/archive/identwin.htm>.

A New Perspective

When we accurately consider how variables can affect research, we gain a different perception of the challenges faced by nutritional scientists. It then becomes clear that the nutrition industry demands a more open perspective than, for example, the car racing industry. In car racing there are, of course, variables, many of which are related to breakdowns or improvements affecting performance. These are generally much easier to track down than those related to nutrition, however, due to the fact that specialists thoroughly know the mechanical structures of the vehicles, how to repair them, and how to improve upon them. Unlike the human body, cars don't have genetic histories and we are able to understand the mechanics of how they work at every level. All in all, there are simply less variables to consider.

While often compared to a car in nutrition-related examples, the human body is unquestionably far more complex. For simplistic examples, however, cars and their care provide some useful analogies. A car with too little oil or gas won't get us very far. A body with a severe deficiency of water or nutrients isn't likely to either. In each case an equilibrium is disrupted. Similarly, adding small amounts of combined detrimental substances to a car's gas tank on a regular basis can be compared to consistently ingesting foods that contain small amounts of combined chemical additives and pesticide residues. Somewhere down the line one or more problems are likely to arise.

An Awareness We Can Use

Becoming aware of nutrition-related variables not only gives us insight into why nutrition is confusing, but also provides us with a tool that can be used to make worthwhile nutritional choices. Once we have the ability to recognize the variables associated with specific foods and food products we can research their effects and more readily learn what's best to consume. It is this approach that enables us to see past the confusion and develop a better understanding of nutrition. In chapter two we build on this concept by taking a more complete look at choice-related variables and how we can use them to our benefit.

Chapter 2

*W*hile variables often cause nutrition to be confusing, they also play an essential role in making sense of it. Becoming familiar with the specific variable options associated with the development of individual foods and food-related products and learning how to gather the most accurate information about them are the keys to developing a clearer understanding of what's best to consume. Through these beneficial efforts we become better equipped to make conscientious, well-informed nutritional choices and are more capable of establishing the most effective nutritional strategies for optimal health. The process is relatively simple and can successfully be put into action in spite of the fact that we are constantly inundated with new information and varying opinions about how foods, nutrients, and additives affect us.

The easiest and most effective way to begin is to consider foods, beverages, and other consumables as main "surface" variables, and anything associated with their production, consumption, and experimentation as sub-variables. For example, if a tomato is our main variable, the sub-variables involved will include how it was grown (e.g., conventionally, organically, in soil, hydroponically, aeroponically), the types of treatment it underwent (e.g., pesticides, fertilizers, genetic modification, irradiation, gassing), and the types of nutritional benefits it will provide (e.g., vitamins, minerals, antioxidants, fiber), among other things.

Next it is essential to recognize that most main variables have different sub-variables. Even apples do not have sub-variables identical to those of bananas, even though both are fruits. For example, bananas are often treated with ethylene gas to promote ripening, while apples are not. While many main variables have factors in common, they often have distinct differences in production and nutrient content. Becoming familiar with the sub-variables that are unique to each main variable is an important step in making accurate assessments about how foods and products can affect our health.

Finally, we need to know how and where to find the most reliable information about food-related topics. Comparing research from top colleges and other respected sources that specialize in nutrition generally provides the most efficient overview. This doesn't mean that every other avenue from which we can gather knowledge about nutrition is worthless; on the contrary, it gives us a base from which to compare and investigate *all* information so that we may learn to make informed choices based on facts. It also doesn't mean that the information from colleges and other dependable sources is exempt from error or a lack of information, as there will always be some level of uncertainty in nutrition due to the high ratio of variable activity. The bottom line is that reviewing information directly from more than one main research source is best, and getting that information from credible sources is vital. Acquiring the most current data is also essential in most cases, though consulting past research often has value as well, especially when different issues related to the same topic were previously investigated. Care must be taken however, especially when using the internet, to ensure that the information being retrieved is indeed from the source we are seeking. Many authorities also advise against solely considering the results of tests funded by corporations or other entities that have an interest in the food or product being tested.

Obtaining the information in a consumer-friendly format is also a priority. Most colleges and universities provide summaries of experiments on consumables that are relatively easy to understand and from which we can develop our own perspectives. Easy-to-read material is also available from the U.S. Food and Drug Administration (FDA), the U.S. Department of Agriculture (USDA), the National Institutes of Health (NIH), and the U.S. Environmental Protection Agency (EPA). These governmental agencies coordinate with each other in addition to working with a wide array of researchers, many of whom are from the college and university sector. Even the media presents a variety of avenues for learning about nutrition. However, due to time restraints and other factors, news clips generally don't provide too many specifics. For example, when we are told that coffee has certain health attributes, we may not be informed as to what type of coffee was tested, where it was from, and whether or not all coffees provide the same benefits. In cases like this we can gain additional clarity by reviewing the information directly from the researcher or research group that performed the testing.

Overall, there are three things we can do to effectively obtain information about what we consume:

1. **Review the Research.** Looking up variables and general nutritional information, especially about foods and related products that are consumed regularly, gives us a clearer idea about how what we consume affects our health. This should be done periodically to keep up with new information. Keeping a notebook is helpful.

2. **Read Labels and Signs.** Learning what is and isn't in foods and related products and finding out some of the treatments they've undergone can be accomplished by reading what's written on the packaging, or, in the case of produce or seafood, what's written on packaging or any signs that may be available. This is especially important with foods consumed on a regular basis. Also keep in mind that ingredients and production methods, and therefore labels and signs, often change. Re-reading them on occasion helps us stay alert to changes.

3. **Ask the Source.** If there is uncertainty about a food or other consumable even after reading a label or sign and gathering any available research, we can consult the supplier, producer, or manufacturer for additional information. If the information they provide is incomplete, evasive, questionable, or doesn't otherwise provide the answers we are looking for, we have the option of finding another source from which to obtain the food or product, or choosing another food or product altogether. In restaurant settings, chefs

and food managers are often quite knowledgeable about the foods being prepared and usually don't mind being asked about them.

Once we recognize the various types of sub-variables associated with what we consume and can effectively gather facts about them, much of the mystery about nutrition—and therefore much of the confusion—is alleviated. We can then successfully steer through the effects of variable activity and develop our nutritional perspectives with greater accuracy.

Putting Variables Into Action

Grouping sub-variables together with their main variables allows us to see the developmental and nutritional aspects involved with specific foods and food-related products. The next step is to research any issues that are of concern to us prior to making hands-on nutritional choices. This process affords us the opportunity to use variables as a blueprint for improving our diets. In effect, we learn how to put their power into practical daily use rather than being confused by them.

The remainder of this chapter presents a number of common main variables along with many of their sub-variables, as well as suggestions for healthful choices. Note that the use of certified 100% organic foods and products, or those that have been produced in a similar or better manner (such as those that are home grown in nutrient-filled soil without pesticides) is frequently recommended (see chapter ten for more information on organics). This is based on the idea that the less a food is manipulated and the less pesticides, antibiotics, hormones, or other chemicals it is exposed to, the better. Our bodies must process each of these to get rid of them, and many have residual effects, an issue of particular concern with regard to children, the elderly, and those who are ill. Another important consideration is that while the amounts of chemicals found in foods often fall within allowable limits set by regulatory agencies, their effects when combined are largely unknown.

Foods

Meat

There are conventional, organic, and wild-caught meats. They are available in many different forms from fresh to freeze-dried and come from a variety of animals including cows, deer, lambs, and buffalo. All are high in protein; most are high in zinc, iron, and B vitamins as well. Among them, beef is the most commonly consumed. In 2004 alone the total estimated U.S. consumption of beef was 27.8 billion pounds.[1]

Most meats are categorized by cut alone or by both cut and grade (the exceptions are liver and other organ meats, which are categorized separately). Cuts include steaks, chops, ribs, and roasts. Grades are used to indicate the quality of cuts in terms of tenderness, juiciness, and flavor. Lower-grade cuts are derived from actively used muscle areas such as the shoulders, flanks, and legs, and are generally less tender than other cuts. Higher-grade cuts are from less-used muscle areas such as the rib and loin sections. These contain more flecks of fat throughout their lean areas, which is referred to as marbling. This creates a greater degree of tenderness and juiciness as well as heightened flavor.

Beef, veal, lamb, and mutton are all graded for retail sales. Pork is also graded, though not at the consumer level. Beef is the most graded of all meats, with a total of eight USDA grades: Prime, Choice, Select, Standard, Commercial, Utility, Cutter, and Canner. USDA Choice is the most widely sold grade. USDA Prime, Choice, Select, and Standard grades are derived from younger animals. Standard and Commercial grade beef is often sold ungraded. The three lower grades, USDA Utility, Cutter, and Canner, are not generally sold individually, but rather are used to make ground beef, hot dogs, and other meat products.

Ground meats are derived from one animal, from several animals of the same type, or from a combination of two or more distinctly different types

---

[1] United States Department of Agriculture, Economic Research Service, July 7, 2005, <http://www.ers.usda.gov/news/BSECoverage.htm> (March 8, 2006).

of animals, such as occurs with beef and pork mixtures used to create sausage. Among beef selections, hamburger and fabricated beef steaks are permitted to have additional fat added during production, while ground and chopped beef are not.[2]

Conventional meats are permitted to undergo irradiation in order to destroy pathogens, but must then be labeled or otherwise designated as such. Organic meats are not permitted to be irradiated.

BEST CHOICE: Fresh, lean cuts of certified 100% organic meat or meat produced in a similar or better manner.

CONSIDERATIONS: Conventional meats can contain hormones, antibiotics, pesticides, or other chemicals, or any combination of these, or the animals from which these meats are derived may have been previously exposed to such chemicals. Wild-caught meats are less likely to contain hormones or antibiotics, though they may contain pesticides or other chemicals depending on the animal's diet and various environmental factors. Organic meats are obtained from animals that have been raised without hormones or antibiotics and have been continuously fed certified 100% organic feed.

Some meats are naturally or artificially treated to maintain or enhance their color, flavor, or both. This is typical of many processed conventional meats, including those sold in bulk. In addition to color and flavor enhancers, many conventional meat products contain fillers and chemical preservatives.

Poultry
Among the options in this category are chicken, duck, goose, and turkey, and somewhat less common selections such as ostrich, quail, and pheasant. There are both conventionally raised and organic varieties from which to choose, along with their wild-caught counterparts. We can select from fresh natural poultry that has undergone minimal processing and contains no

---

[2] United States Department of Agriculture, Food Safety & Inspection Service, *Code of Federal Regulations.* Title 9, Volume 2, p. 298-299, 9CFR319.15 Washington: GPO, January 2003.

added ingredients, or frozen, canned, and packaged poultry prepared with solutions that contain varying amounts of water, salt, flavor enhancers, phosphates, and other ingredients. Conventional poultry is permitted to be irradiated, but must then be labeled or otherwise designated as such. U.S. consumption of poultry meat (broilers, other chicken, turkey) is considerably higher than either beef or pork, but less than total red meat consumption.[3] Chicken is the number one species consumed by Americans.[4]

BEST CHOICE: Fresh or fresh-frozen certified 100% organic free-range birds that have undergone minimal processing or those that have been produced in a manner that is similar or better.

CONSIDERATIONS: No hormones are permitted to be used when raising poultry, though antibiotics and pesticides are often used in the production of birds that are not organic. Conventional poultry may also be given feed that has been produced with the use of pesticides, herbicides, fungicides, or other chemicals, or any combination of these, and may contain residues of them. Wild-caught poultry may also contain or have been exposed to such chemicals.

Fish & Seafood
Like beef and poultry, fish is available in many different forms including fresh, smoked, pickled, and dried. It is permitted to be irradiated so long as it is properly labeled or designated as such. We can choose from freshwater species such as cod and haddock or saltwater varieties including snapper, grouper, and sea bass. There is also an abundance of shellfish and other seafood from which to choose. Both fish and shellfish are available wild caught or farm-raised. Farm-raised selections include catfish (highest in sales), trout, salmon, tilapia, hybrid striped bass, sturgeon, walleye, and yellow

---

[3] United States Department of Agriculture, Economic Research Service, August 2005, <http://www.ers.usda.gov/Briefing/Poultry/> (March 11, 2006).
[4] United States Department of Agriculture, Food Safety & Inspection Service, Feb. 2003, <http://www.fsis.usda.gov/Fact_Sheets/Chicken_Food_Safety_Focus/index.asp> (March 7, 2006).

perch, and a variety of mollusks including oysters, clams, and mussels.[5] Farmed fish and shellfish are often treated with antibiotics; farmed salmon is often fed color-enhancing feed. Although some farmed fish and shellfish are labeled organic, neither is certified as organic by the U.S. government because federal regulations don't yet include organic provisions for fish and seafood. Frozen, previously frozen, canned, and packaged seafood often contains phosphates and sulfites for moisture and color retention, respectively, accounting for other considerations and choices. Fresh seafood is also often treated with sulfites.

BEST CHOICE: Fresh, untreated wild-caught seafood from unpolluted waters.

CONSIDERATIONS: Mercury intake from fish can cause health concerns, especially for children, women who are pregnant or nursing, and women in their childbearing years who may become pregnant. Fish that are generally high in mercury include shark, swordfish, tilefish, king mackerel, and some species of fresh or frozen tuna; low-mercury fish include salmon, catfish, and freshwater trout. A more complete list can be accessed on the Natural Resources Defense Council website at **http://www.nrdc.org/ health/effects/mercury/guide.asp**. The FDA and other sources also provide information on mercury content in seafood. It should be noted that each listing may contain different information due to the size of the fish tested and the location and condition of the waters from which they were taken, among other factors. Reports on the condition of various bodies of water can be accessed at **www.epa.gov**. Public health departments also provide local advisories. Fish should be skinned and their organs removed prior to cooking to reduce the potential for ingesting contaminants. Overall, smaller species generally contain less mercury.

---

[5] United States Department of Agriculture, Economic Research Service, March 2, 2005, <http://www.ers.usda.gov/Briefing/Aquaculture/background.htm> (Dec. 8, 2007).

Eggs

Common egg selections include those from chickens, ducks, and quail. We can choose from organic or conventional varieties as well as those obtained from caged, cage-free, or free-range animals. We can also choose them based on size, grade, nutrient content, and color. Chicken eggs are generally either white or brown. This is determined by breed and is indicated by the hue of a hen's earlobes.[6] It has no bearing on nutritional content. Although they are rarer in the U.S., certain breeds also produce eggs in hues of blue, green, and other colors. Per capita egg consumption in 2004, based on data for both eggs and processed egg products, was approximately 256 eggs, an increase of 21 eggs per person compared to a decade ago.[7]

BEST CHOICE: Fresh eggs from certified 100% organically raised free-range chickens or those produced in a manner that is similar or better.

CONSIDERATIONS: Eggs contain every vitamin except vitamin C. Their cholesterol is found solely in the yolk. One large Grade A egg has between approximately 180 and 215 milligrams of cholesterol. Although cholesterol from eggs may not be as detrimental to the body as once thought, ways to reduce the cholesterol content in eggs are currently being investigated. Eggs are freshest when their whites are cloudy and less fresh when their whites are clear.[8] The harder a hard-boiled egg is to peel, the fresher it is.[9] Eggs from conventionally raised poultry may be exposed to pesticides and other chemicals. According to the EPA, pesticide residues may enter eggs when pesticides are present in the feed of hens or when

---

[6] Latour, Mickey A., "Nomenclature, Eggs & Tidbits of Information," Purdue University, n.d., <http://ag.ansc.purdue.edu/poultry/chickzone/geninfo.htm>. (March 22, 2006).
[7] United States Dept. of Agriculture, ERS, December 2005, <http://www.ers.usda.gov/data/foodconsumption/spreadsheets/eggs.xls#eggspcc!a1> (March 11, 2006).
[8] United States Dept. of Agriculture, Food Safety & Inspection Service, Feb. 2003, <http://www.fsis.usda.gov/Fact_Sheets/Focus_On_Shell_Eggs/index.asp> (November 8, 2006).
[9] See footnote 8.

hens are directly treated with pesticides for external parasites.[10] Conventionally produced fresh shell eggs are permitted to be irradiated as long as they are correctly labeled or otherwise designated as such.

Dairy Foods

Among dairy food choices are hard cheeses such as cheddar, mozzarella, and Colby, soft cheeses including ricotta, cottage cheese, and cream cheese, and processed cheeses such as American and artificial Swiss. Other choices include yogurt, pudding, ice cream, and butter. Low-fat, reduced fat, nonfat, lactose-free, lactose-reduced, low-sodium, and sodium-free versions are available for many of these foods. We can select from conventional or organic types, including those made with or without added colors, flavors, preservatives, or other additives. Our options include products produced from cow's milk or the milk of sheep, goats, or other animals. There are also products made from raw milk. In 2004, Americans consumed an average of 31.3 pounds of whole and part-skim milk cheese and 23.2 pounds of regular and low-fat ice cream per person, all from cow's milk alone.[11]

BEST CHOICE: Fresh, low-fat, certified 100% organic products or those produced in a similar or better manner. Products should also be lactose-reduced or lactose-free and low-sodium or sodium-free as required.

CONSIDERATIONS: Like conventional meats, conventional dairy products can contain residues from hormones, antibiotics, pesticides, or other chemicals, or any combination of these. Because such chemicals harbor themselves in fat, conventionally produced butter, cheese, ice cream, and other high-fat foods are at risk for higher levels of residues. Low-fat choices are healthier overall. The use of lactose-free products is beneficial for those

[10] Podhorniak, Lynda V., et al., "A Collaborative Effort Between the U.S. Environmental Protection Agency, the Food and Drug Administration, and the University of Arkansas to Develop a Method for the Determination of Part Per Billion Levels of Carbamate Pesticide Residues in Eggs," 2005, *EPA Science Forum*.
[11] United States Dept. of Agriculture, Economic Research Service, December 21, 2005, <http://www.ers.usda.gov/Data/FoodConsumption/spreadsheets/dymfg.xls#AllDairyPcc!a1> (May 2, 2006).

who lack the lactase enzyme and have difficulty digesting milk-based products. Between 30 and 50 million Americans are affected by this condition, which is known as lactose intolerance.[12]

Nuts & Seeds

We can choose from nuts and edible seeds that are raw, dry roasted, or roasted in a variety of oils including peanut and cottonseed oil. We can also select them in the form of nut butters and as part of numerous salads, candies, cereals, baked goods, and prepared dishes. Many are treated with seasonings, preservatives, and artificial colors. Those that are conventionally produced may contain residues from pesticides, herbicides, fungicides, rodenticides, or other chemicals, or any combination of these. The top three most consumed nuts in the U.S. are almonds, walnuts, and pecans.[13] Other choices include:

Hazelnuts (Filberts)	Brazil nuts
Cashews	Pumpkin seeds
Macadamia nuts	Peanuts (actually a legume)
Pistachios	Sunflower seeds
Pine nuts (pignolis)	Sesame seeds

BEST CHOICE: Fresh, raw, certified 100% organic nuts or those produced in a similar or better manner.

CONSIDERATIONS: Hazelnuts (filberts) and sunflower seeds contain the highest ratio of nutrients per serving.

Those who have dental problems or intestinal disorders and are unable to chew or digest nuts may benefit from well-blended nut butters.

---

[12] NDDIC, "Lactose intolerance," *NIH Publication No. 06–2751*, March 2006,
<http://digestive.niddk.nih.gov/ddiseases/pubs/lactoseintolerance/> November 8, 2006.
[13] United States Dept. of Agriculture, Economic Research Service, October 8, 2004,
<http://www.ers.usda.gov/Briefing/FruitAndTreeNuts/background.htm> (March 11, 2006).

Rancid nuts should be avoided, as their oils contain chemicals that can damage cells and may promote cholesterol to clog the arteries. An unpleasant odor and off taste are characteristic signs of rancidity.[14]

Grains

Grain food selections include those that contain whole or refined grains or a combination of the two. Whole grains have the bran, germ, and endosperm included, and are rich in fiber and nutrients. Among them are wheat, barley, rye, cracked wheat (bulgur), oatmeal, cornmeal, and brown rice, and less well known grains such as kamut, amaranth, millet, quinoa, and triticale. In contrast, refined grains usually contain no bran or germ and are deficient in fiber, iron, and B vitamins, each of which may be replaced in a different form. For example, soy fiber is sometimes added to refined wheat flour during bread production rather than the grain's own natural fiber. Refined grain food choices include white bread (including many types that claim to be whole wheat), crackers, pasta, white rice, farina, and degermed cornmeal. Refined products often undergo bleaching processes and contain a number of additives, creating other considerations.

BEST CHOICE: Certified 100% organic whole grain products or those produced in a similar or better manner.

CONSIDERATIONS: Conventionally produced grains are often exposed to pesticides, herbicides, fungicides, and rodenticides, and may contain residual amounts of one or more of these. The majority of the wheat samples tested as part of the USDA Pesticide Data Program in 2005 contained pesticide residues.[15]

Those who have grain allergies and digestive ailments and need to avoid whole grains or specific types of grain may benefit from specialty replacement products.

---

[14] Kendall, P. and Rausch, J., "Flavored Vinegars and Oils," *No. 9.340,* Colorado State Univ. Cooperative Extension, June 2006, <http://www.ext.colostate.edu/Pubs/foodnut/09340.html> (November 8, 2006).
[15] United States Dept. of Agriculture, AMS, Pesticide Data Program, November 2006. <http://www.ams.usda.gov/Science/pdp/Summary2005.pdf> (November 8, 2006).

Fruit

Fruit can be obtained fresh, frozen, or dried, and as part of candies, baked goods, sauces, and prepared foods. Both conventional and organic varieties are available. Conventional types may be genetically modified or irradiated; if irradiated they must be labeled or otherwise designated as such. They may also have been exposed to pesticides, herbicides, fungicides, or rodenticides, or a variety of other chemicals, and may contain residues of one or more of them. Some fresh fruits, both conventional and organic, may be gassed to hasten ripening. This includes bananas, tomatoes, and avocados. There are dozens of common fruits and thousands of varieties to choose from. Oranges are the most consumed fruit in the U.S., with grapes, apples, bananas, and grapefruit also being high in consumption.[16,17]

BEST CHOICE: Fresh certified 100% organic fruit or fruit that has been produced in a similar or better manner.

CONSIDERATIONS: According to data from the 2005 USDA Pesticide Data Program Annual Summary, apples, grapes, and strawberries contained the highest ratios of pesticide residues among the fresh fruits tested, while watermelon had the least.[18]

Raw fruits are generally highest in nutritional value. Cutting, cooking, soaking, and storage deplete their nutrients. However, in some cases, such as with lycopene in tomatoes, cooking can actually increase nutrient availability.[19]

Baked, poached, or sautéed fruits are often useful for those who have difficulty chewing them or digesting them raw, as well as for chemotherapy patients who are required to avoid raw foods.

---

[16] Perez, A. and Pollack, S., United States Dept. of Agriculture, ERS, *Fruit and Tree Nuts Outlook, FTS-296,* January 31, 2002, < http://www.ers.usda.gov/publications/fts/jan02/fts296.pdf > (March 11, 2006).
[17] United States Dept. of Agriculture, Economic Research Service, February 24, 2009, <http://www.ers.usda.gov/Briefing/FruitAndTreeNuts/background.htm> (April 27, 2009).
[18] United States Dept. of Agriculture, Agricultural Marketing Service, November 2006, <http://www.ams.usda.gov/Science/pdp/Summary2005.pdf> (November 8, 2006).
[19] The Trustees of Indiana University, "Cooked Tomatoes Are Better Than Raw Ones?" Aug. 13, 2002, *A Moment of Science,*® <http://amos.indiana.edu/library/scripts/cooktomato.html> (March 14, 2007).

Vegetables

Like fruits, vegetables can be obtained fresh, frozen, or dried, and as part of baked goods, sauces, and prepared foods, including snacks. Both conventional and organic varieties are available. Conventional types are permitted to be genetically modified or irradiated, though when irradiated they must be labeled or otherwise designated as such. Some vegetables, of both conventional and organic origin, are subject to treatment with ethylene gas to speed ripening.

Among our overall vegetable choices are cruciferous vegetables such as broccoli and cauliflower, nightshade vegetables including green peppers and eggplant, and a variety of legumes in the form of beans and peas. Potatoes, corn, and onions are among those with the highest consumption in the United States.[20]

BEST CHOICE: Fresh, raw, certified 100% organic vegetables or those that have been produced in a similar or better manner.

CONSIDERATIONS: Similar to other crop-based foods, vegetables may be exposed to pesticides, herbicides, fungicides, or rodenticides, or a variety of other chemicals, and may contain residues of one or more of them. According to data from the 2005 USDA Pesticide Data Program Annual Summary, lettuce and cauliflower contained the highest ratios of pesticide residues among the fresh vegetables tested, while green beans and eggplant had the least. Out of the 743 lettuce samples tested, 43 different pesticide residues were found.[21] Data from the program's 2004 Annual Summary also showed a high ratio of residues in the sweet bell peppers tested.[22]

As with fruits, raw vegetables generally have the most nutritional value. Cutting, cooking, soaking, and storage usually deplete their nutrients. Specific

[20] U.S. Dept. of Agriculture, Economic Research Service, Dec. 21, 2005, <http://www.ers.usda.gov/Data/FoodConsumption/spreadsheets/vegtot.xls#Total!a1> (March 11, 2006).
[21] U.S. Dept. of Agriculture, Agr .Marketing Service, November 2006, <http://www.ams.usda.gov/Science/ pdp/Summary2005.pdf> (November 8, 2006).
[22] U.S. Dept. of Agriculture, Agr. Marketing Service, February 2006, <http:// www.ams.usda.gov/Science/pdp/Summary2004.pdf> (November 8, 2006).

methods of cooking certain vegetables, however, may be an exception, though more research is needed in this area. Steamed vegetables that are not overcooked are often a good option for those who have difficulty chewing them or digesting them raw, as well as for chemotherapy patients who are required to avoid raw foods.

Oils

We can choose from oils derived from nuts (almond, macadamia), seeds (coconut, sunflower), legumes (peanut), fruits (olive, avocado), fish (salmon), cows (butter oil), rice, and even algae.[23] We can choose them according to taste, nutritional value, and fat content. There are both conventional and organic types; those that are conventional may or may not be produced from genetically modified foods. (Genetically modified oils include "high oleic" canola, sunflower, and safflower oils, which have been designed to be high in monounsaturated fats. See chapter six for more information on types of fats). Conventionally produced oils are also permitted to be obtained from irradiated foods but must be labeled or otherwise designated as such. Some oils are available unrefined; many, however, undergo filtering, bleaching, and deodorizing processes. This includes oils used in margarines and spreads. Cost is an additional choice factor. Pure, unrefined, first cold pressed olive oils, for example, can be as much as $100 or more per bottle. The major U.S. oilseed crops are soybeans, cottonseeds, canola, rapeseeds, sunflower seeds, and peanuts. Soybeans are the dominant oilseed in the U.S., accounting for about 90 percent of U.S. oilseed production.[24]

BEST CHOICE: Fresh, certified 100% organic oils that are unrefined and first cold pressed (derived from the first pressing of the olives without the use of heat, which can cause nutrient loss) or those that have been produced

---

[23] U.S. Dept. of Agriculture, ARS, "A Link in the Chain: From Oil Refinement to Baby Formula," March 14, 2006, <http://www.ars.usda.gov/is/AR/archive/dec02/oil1202.htm?pf=1> (March 15, 2006).
[24] U.S. Dept. of Agriculture, Economic Research Service, April 25, 2005, <http://www.ers.usda.gov/Briefing/SoybeansOilCrops/background.htm> (March 13, 2006).

in a similar or better manner. Among olive oils, those that are unrefined, extra virgin, and first cold pressed are preferable, as they are generally of the highest overall quality.

CONSIDERATIONS: As with nuts and seeds, oils should be checked for rancidity (the development of an undesirable odor and flavor are good indicators that an oil has become rancid). Conventionally produced oils may contain residues from pesticides, fungicides, herbicides, or other chemicals, or any combination of these.

Herbs & Spices

As common counterparts to foods, herbs and spices are used mainly for taste and color enhancement. Some are also used as preservatives. Many have health benefits or require health precautions, or both. There are both conventional and organic types. Those that are conventionally produced may be irradiated, particularly if sold commercially or used in commercial products, though they must be labeled or otherwise designated as such. Vanilla (which is derived from a specific variety of orchid) and saffron are the most expensive among spices.

BEST CHOICE: Certified 100% organic herbs and spices or those that have been produced in a similar or better manner.

CONSIDERATIONS: Those taking medication should become aware of and avoid any drug interactions with herbs and spices. Like other crop-based plants, conventionally produced herbs and spices that have been treated with pesticides, fungicides, herbicides, or other chemicals may contain residues of one or more of these.

Now let's take a look at choice-related variables involving what we drink.

Beverages

Water

Water comes in many forms and is derived from a wide variety of sources extending well beyond the tap. The variables that affect it include location and method of extraction; temperature; mineral and element content; and exposure to microorganisms. When bottled, it is part of a large and growing market segment, ranking second among commercial beverage categories by volume just behind carbonated soft drinks.[25] In 2005 the national per capita average was 26.1 gallons per person.[26]

There are hundreds of brands of bottled water in the U.S. Some are imported. Some are enhanced. Some are simply municipal water bottled for sale. The different types that are available include:

- purified water
- spring water
- distilled water
- well water
- artesian water
- artesian well water
- tonic water
- soda water
- sterilized water
- reverse osmosis water
- mineral water
- natural sparkling mineral water
- water enhanced with minerals
- water with the minerals removed
- flavored water
- water with caffeine
- sports or fitness water
- sparkling water

BEST CHOICE: Clean, uncontaminated natural water that meets or beats both the EPA's drinking water standards and the World Health Organization's guidelines for drinking water quality.

---

[25] "Bottled Water Strengthens Position As No. 2 Beverage," April 25, 2005, <http://www.beverage marketing.com> (November 20, 2006).
[26] "Bottled Water Continues Tradition of Strong Growth in 2005," April 2006, <http://www.beveragemarketing.com> (November 20, 2006).

CONSIDERATIONS: While science has yet to prove that any one particular type or brand of water is ideal for the human body, consuming water that is free of chemicals and pathogens is a priority for many of us. Overall, clean water that is low in total dissolved solids (including minerals, salts, metals, and other substances) appears to be a safe bet. While properly functioning distillation units and reverse osmosis systems with added carbon filtration can reduce or eliminate a variety of chemicals and pathogens that are often found in other forms of drinking water, they must be well maintained in order to avoid bacterial buildup. Also, the water created by these systems is demineralized, meaning that it does not contain minerals needed for good health. This type of water may even leach nutrients from foods during cooking. Adding low levels of appropriate liquid minerals to demineralized water may be beneficial.

Soft Drinks

Soft drinks present other beverage choices. Carbonated versions are the top consumer selection among those sold commercially, though estimated per capita consumption actually dropped to 53.7 gallons in 2004 from 54.5 gallons in 2000.[27] There are hundreds of different types of carbonated drinks and numerous formulations, including those created with or without caffeine, sugar, carbs, calories, or sodium. Many contain a variety of sugars or artificial sweeteners, or a mixture of the two, and any number of additives to enhance color, taste, aroma, and shelf life. Some also have added nutrients or herbs. In 2005 Americans consumed an average of 52.9 gallons per person.[28]

Non-carbonated soft drinks are available in canned, bottled, packaged, or powdered form and include fruit-flavored beverages such as lemonade, fruit punch, and tea. Most consist mainly of water combined with one or more forms of sugar and a variety of additives including colors, flavors, and

---

[27] "U.S. Soft Drink Sales Up Slightly in 2004," March 14, 2005, <http://www.beveragemarketing.com> (November 20, 2006).
[28] "Carbonated Soft Drinks Suffer Setback in 2005," April 2006, <http://www.beveragemarketing.com> (November 20, 2006).

preservatives. They may or may not contain any real fruit. Some have added herbs or nutrients.

BEST CHOICE: Organic soft drinks or those that have been produced in a similar or better manner. Those with lower sugar content are preferable.

CONSIDERATIONS: According to a study published in the American Journal of Clinical Nutrition, the consumption of carbonated cola beverages by women may be a risk factor for developing low bone mineral density.[29] Most non-diet soft drinks are high in sugar. The ingredients used in the production of any particular soft drink may differ depending on how it is dispensed.

Coffee

Coffee comes in many forms from fresh ground to freeze-dried and is derived from a number of countries. There are hot and iced varieties of regular roast, specialty, and gourmet coffees, including espresso, cappuccino, latte, and other creations. (Arabica and Robusta are the two types of coffee beans predominantly used in the coffee industry.) Many coffees contain caffeine, while others are decaffeinated or caffeine free. The amount of caffeine in regular and decaffeinated coffees can vary widely. Decaffeinated coffees generally retain at least a small amount of caffeine after processing, though some provide a larger dose.[30] Additionally, the fact that one coffee produces a darker brew than another does not necessarily mean it is higher in caffeine.

Sugars, syrups, artificial sweeteners, and a variety of dairy and non-dairy products are options for enhancing coffee taste. Coffee brands, types, and levels of quality provide us with other choices. According to the National

---

[29] Tucker, K.L, et al., "Colas, but not other carbonated beverages, are associated with low bone mineral density in older women: The Framingham Osteoporosis Study," *American Journal of Clinical Nutrition,* Vol. 84, No. 4, 936-942, Oct. 2006, <http://www.ajcn.org/cgi/content/abstract/84/4/936>.

[30] Nordlie, Tom, "UF study finds specialty coffee's caffeine content capricious," *University of Florida News,* October 10, 2006, < http://news.ufl.edu/2006/10/10/decaf/> (March 27, 2006).

Coffee Association of the U.S.A., over 121 million people in the nation drink coffee every day.[31]

BEST CHOICE: Fresh, 100% certified organic coffee or that which has been produced in a similar or better manner.

CONSIDERATIONS: Like other conventional crops, conventionally produced coffee is often treated with pesticides, fungicides, herbicides, and other chemicals and may contain residues of one or more of them.

Tea

Tea also holds a position among the top beverage picks. Like coffee, it is harvested in several countries, comes in numerous flavors, and can be served hot or iced with a variety of flavor enhancers. Both conventional and organic types are available. When conventionally produced it may contain residues from pesticides, fungicides, herbicides, and other chemicals, or any combination of these. We can select from leaf teas made strictly from leaves, or herbal teas made from any combination of leaves, flowers, berries, roots, stems, and bark. Both herbal and standard commercial teas can be obtained with or without caffeine. Green tea currently accounts for a growing segment of the tea industry.

BEST CHOICE: Fresh, 100% certified organic tea or that which has been produced in a similar or better manner. Unbleached tea bags are preferable among bagged teas.

CONSIDERATIONS: Unlike standard commercial teas, herbal teas usually contain no theobromine (a central nervous system stimulant similar to caffeine) and many are known to have health benefits. However, some herbal teas and herbal tea products can cause illness or death if used improperly.

---

[31] "National Coffee Drinking Trends," National Coffee Association of U.S.A., Inc., 2006, <www.ncausa.org>.

Infants should not be given herbal teas unless specifically recommended and carefully monitored by a qualified physician. Those taking any type of medication should become aware of and avoid all teas with ingredients that cause negative food and drug interactions. This can be done by contacting the prescribing physician, pharmacists, and the drug manufacturer.

Alcoholic Beverages

Taste, quality, alcohol content, ingredients, and processing methods each account for choices when selecting alcoholic drinks. Product age is also a common factor. Selections include beer, wine, and distilled spirits. Some are available in organic form. Commercial beer choices include those that are either light or dark in color, mild or robust in flavor, and high or low in carbohydrates and calories. They may be made with hops or a variety of other ingredients including honey, molasses, and fruit. There are lagers, ales, and steam beers, and their close relatives, malt liquors (higher alcohol content than beer) and malt beverages (lower alcohol content than beer). They may be domestic or imported. Malt beverages are usually fruit flavored and often contain high amounts of sugar in the form of corn syrup.

Wine is available made from numerous varieties of grapes obtained from different vineyards throughout the world. It is also available made from honey and a variety of fruits other than grapes, including cherries, raspberries, blueberries, pineapples, and honeydew. It may be slightly or considerably aged. Many wines contain added sulfites (a preservative that approximately 1 in 100 people are allergic to[32]); others are available sulfite-free or contain only naturally occurring sulfites.

Distilled spirits, including rum, vodka, and whiskey, are also available domestically as well as from other countries and can undergo a variety of processing methods. Rum is available in different types made from sugar cane or molasses; vodka is made mainly from cereal grains including wheat, barley, and rye (though it can also be made from potatoes or beets); and

---

[32] Papazian, Ruth, "Sulfites: Safe for Most, Dangerous for Some," December 1996, <http://www.fda.gov/fdac/features/096_sulf.html>. (March 27, 2006).

whiskey is usually produced from corn, rye, wheat, barley, or other grains, or some combination thereof.[33] These beverages often differ in taste and color and may be consumed alone or mixed in any of hundreds of combinations using variable ingredients such as fruit, cream, coffee, spices, and flavorings.

BEST CHOICE: 100% certified organic alcoholic beverages or those that have been produced in a similar or better manner.

CONSIDERATIONS: When alcohol is ingested it breaks down and releases a number of toxic substances into the bloodstream. As a result, all alcoholic beverages have detrimental effects on the body. While some research shows potential benefits from occasional or even daily consumption of specific types and amounts of alcoholic beverages, health problems can be incurred at the same time. A benefit to the heart from wine consumption, for example, may be overridden by the potential for liver disease, cancer, or, ironically, heart disease or stroke due to alcohol consumption.

Juice

Fruit and vegetable juices can be obtained fresh, frozen, or from concentrate, and may be unpasteurized, pasteurized, ultra pasteurized, or flash pasteurized (see chapter nine, *Food Safety & Technology*, for additional details on pasteurization). They are available with or without added nutrients, made from local fruit, imported fruit, or a combination of the two, and may be organic or conventionally derived. Some are available pulp-free or with varied amounts of pulp. Each juice or juice combination may be derived from non-irradiated, irradiated, or genetically modified fruits or vegetables, or a combination of these, though irradiated versions must be labeled or otherwise designated as such. They may also contain natural or artificial preservatives or coloring agents, or both. Conventional types may be derived from

[33] Beverage Testing Institute, "Rum," <http://www.tastings.com/spirits/rum.html>, "Vodka," <http://www.tastings.com/ spirits/vodka.html>, "North American Whiskey," <http:www.tastings.com/spirits/American_whiskey.html> (March 27, 2006).

fruits or vegetables that have been exposed to pesticides, herbicides, fungicides, or rodenticides, or some combination of these chemicals, and may contain residues of one or more of them.

BEST CHOICE: Fresh squeezed, 100% certified organic juice or that which has been produced in a similar or better manner.

CONSIDERATIONS: Many juices are high in natural sugar. Diluting them with water and drinking them slowly rather than gulping them can be beneficial, as it causes a smaller rise in blood sugar and less impact on the pancreas. Juices with pulp provide fiber which offers additional health benefits. Juice beverages should be checked for their percentage of actual fruit juice content. Heavily sugared beverages with very small amounts of actual fruit juice generally offer less overall nutritional support for the body.

Milk
Milk is obtained mainly from cows, goats, and sheep. Its production often includes the addition of nutrients, namely vitamins A and D, though several brands also offer versions with added calcium. Some types contain lactobacillus acidophilus and lactobacillus bifidus, two digestive aids known to enhance intestinal health. There are also flavored milks and milk-based drinks such as eggnog, each of which may contain one or more natural or artificial additives, including flavorings, colors, and preservatives. Most milk is available from both conventional and organic sources and comes in several or all of the following forms:

- raw
- soured
- unpasteurized
- pasteurized
- flash pasteurized
- ultra pasteurized
- ultra heat-treated (UHT)
- whole
- buttermilk (cultured)
- nonfat powdered or dry
- evaporated
- condensed
- sweetened condensed
- fortified
- fermented
- low-sodium

- low-fat 1%
- low-fat 2%
- nonfat (skim)

- lactose-reduced
- lactose-free
- flavored

Each of these options has the potential to be combined with one or more of the others, providing for additional types. Organic lactose-free 2% low-fat milk, powdered buttermilk, and low-fat milk with acidophilus are examples.

We can also choose from non-dairy versions of milk derived from rice, soy, coconuts, almonds, sesame seeds, and other foods. They too are available from organic or conventional sources, may be flavored or unflavored, and, like fruit juices and dairy milk, may or may not be fortified with additional nutrients. They are often combined with vegetable oils and carrageenan (a seaweed derivative), and in some cases artificial additives. Those that are conventionally produced may contain genetically modified ingredients. They may also be derived from irradiated foods, but must be labeled or otherwise designated as such.

BEST CHOICE: Fresh, low-fat, certified 100% organic products or those produced in a similar or better manner. Products should also be lactose-reduced or lactose-free as required.

CONSIDERATIONS: Similar to conventional meats and dairy foods, conventional milk products can contain residues of hormones, antibiotics, and pesticides, among other chemicals. This is also true of conventionally produced non-dairy milks such as soy milk. In general, lower-fat versions of all types of milk are healthier choices. Raw milk may contain disease-causing bacteria.

Specialty Nutritional Beverages

There are numerous types of sports nutrition beverages and energy and wellness drinks to choose from based on their potential ability to help us acquire specific nutrients, build muscle, enhance hydration, increase stamina, or maintain blood sugar levels. Many are also available for use in losing, gaining, or maintaining weight. Some are medically recommended. Most contain chemical additives including artificial colors and sweeteners. As with many other beverages, conventionally produced versions may contain genetically modified ingredients. They are also permitted to contain irradiated ingredients, though they are required to be labeled or otherwise designated as such when they do. Irradiated products may offer select benefits to those who are ill or have compromised immune systems by reducing the amount of bacteria and other pathogens they contain.

BEST CHOICE: Certified 100% organic products or those produced in a similar or better manner.

CONSIDERATIONS: During illnesses, high quality supplemental liquid nutrition that is additive-free and low in sugar can provide the body with functional support by not requiring it to filter out chemicals or compensate for blood sugar fluctuations. The same holds true for sports drinks and other forms of liquid nutrition. Energy drinks that are high in sugar, caffeine, and stimulant herbs often produce a rebound effect that depletes energy in the long run.

Other Choices

Supplements

There are thousands of nutritional supplements. They include vitamins, minerals, amino acids, and botanicals, including herbs, along with each of their individual constituents. Both naturally derived and chemically produced types are available. We can select from pills, liquids, powders, or chewables. Many contain natural or artificial colors, sweeteners, fillers, and other ingredients. In addition to formulations for children, adults, and the elderly, there are those specifically designed to aid or prevent various medical conditions, such as vitamin C for the prevention of scurvy and folic acid for the prevention of birth defects.

BEST CHOICE: Generally speaking, certified 100% organic food-based products or those produced in a similar or better manner are best, though in some cases this may differ. For example, folic acid (a synthetic version of naturally occurring folate) is better absorbed in the body than folate and may be preferred.

CONSIDERATIONS: Those who consume a nutritious diet and practice other positive lifestyle factors may not require the use of supplements. Those who do require or prefer their use should become well educated about dosages and effects and have regular checkups from a qualified physician. Ingredients in food-based supplements should be carefully reviewed by those with allergies or sensitivities and those taking medication. All types of supplements designed for potential mental or physical enhancement should be carefully researched before use. Conventionally produced food-based supplements have the potential to contain residues from pesticides, herbicides, fungicides, or other chemicals, or any combination of these.

Diets

There are over fifty publicly recognized weight loss diets. Most are based on calorie, carbohydrate, sugar, fat, or protein restriction, while some incorporate more than one of these strategies. Others involve an increase in protein intake or other recommendations. There are also thousands of diet foods and related products, including snacks, cereals, condiments, and candy. Options include foods and beverages made with fat replacements and artificial sweeteners. In 2006 approximately $55.4 billion was spent on weight loss programs and products in the U.S., mainly by American consumers[34] In addition to weight loss regimens there are also a variety of diets designed for weight gain and maintenance.

BEST CHOICE: Varies per individual. Avoid dieting whenever possible.

---

[34] LaRosa, John, "U.S. Weight Loss and Diet Control Market." *Marketdata Enterprises, Inc.* <www.marketdataenterprises.com> April 16, 2007. For further info visit www.bestdietforme.com.

CONSIDERATIONS: Learning how to eat properly and most effectively for our bodies' needs provides lifelong benefits and requires no dieting.

Packaging & Storage Containers

Packaging options include glass, plastic, aluminum, paper, wax paper, paperboard, and steel. There are jars, jugs, bottles, cans, wraps, bags, boxes, bowls, and pouches, among other items, many of which are available from recycled materials. We can choose based on convenience, portability, size, safety, environmental concerns, or a variety of other factors.

The number of convenience-based choices in particular is substantial. Many containers available today are made from materials that are dishwasher, microwave, and oven safe. Some designs offer much versatility, allowing foods to be stored, cooked, and consumed in the same unit.

Choices can also be based on health considerations. While canning and packaging alone frequently affect the color, texture, taste, aroma, and nutrient content of foods and beverages, chemical treatments performed on packaging and storage containers carry the same potential. Most containers undergo one or more processes in which they are coated, colored, sealed, irradiated, or treated with chemicals, including preservatives, though there are also those made from natural, untreated materials. Even without added processing, the basic materials used in the production of containers can directly affect their contents. This is why specific materials are recommended for safe heating and others are not. Many plastic food tubs, for example, are not suitable for microwave use due to their potential to break down and migrate into foods, causing health concerns.

BEST CHOICE: Glass, well-tested approved plastics, and safe, untreated natural materials.

CONSIDERATIONS: Inert materials that don't break down, leach, or otherwise detrimentally affect foods, beverages, and our health are the most beneficial.

Cookware, Tableware & Utensils

The items we use for food preparation and consumption account for other variables. Some of them can directly alter the things we consume. They can be made from a variety of substances including stainless steel, iron, copper, bronze, aluminum, glass, wood, plastic, ceramic, and Teflon.® Many consist of more than one of these materials, such as copper-clad stainless steel, enameled cast iron, and ceramic-coated metals. There are also utensils, mugs, goblets, plates, tea sets, and other items that are made of sterling silver, gold, and other precious elements. Those that generally cause concern are aluminum, ceramics, and iron. The use of aluminum cookware and utensils has raised some apprehension due to the fact that aluminum, which is unnecessary in the body and is known to cause harmful effects, can transfer into foods. The amount ingested in this fashion is thought to be very small, however, in comparison to intake from aluminum-based antacids and buffered aspirin.[35] Anodized aluminum does not appear to carry the same risk. Ceramic cookware and other food-related cooking and storage items that are ceramic often contain lead, sometimes in large quantities, which can leach into foods and cause serious illness or brain damage.[36] Iron ingestion from cookware may present health issues for those who store too much iron in the body.[37]

BEST CHOICE: Glass, high-quality stainless steel, and anodized aluminum.

CONSIDERATIONS: Materials that are inert or otherwise have the least affect on foods, beverages, and our health are preferable.

---

[35] Centers For Disease Control and Prevention, ATSDR, "ToxFAQs™ for Aluminum," June 1999, <http://www.atsdr.cdc.gov/tfacts22.html> (March 15, 2006).
[36] Centers For Disease Control and Prevention, ATSDR, "ToxFAQs™ for Lead," September 2005, <http://www.atsdr.cdc.gov/tfacts13.html> (March 15, 2006).
[37] Weinberg, Eugene D., "Iron Loading and Disease Surveillance," *Emerging Infectious Diseases,* July 1, 1999, <http://www.cdc.gov/ncidod/EID/vol5no3/weinberg.htm> (March 15, 2006).

Convenience Factors

The desire for simple food preparation, or none at all, plays an ever-increasing role in diet. We can select from fast-foods or make foods fast by using quick recipes. In the supermarket, ready-to-eat, prepackaged, and instant products fill shelves and freezers, offering us hundreds of additional options. There are numerous brands and varieties of instant rice, milk, soup, coffee, oats, pasta, and other foods, and one-minute and quick-cooking versions of rice, farina, oats, and pasta, to name a few. There are also various convenience-oriented cooking aids, from fast-rise yeast to self-heating containers. Additionally, microwave and oven-ready foods are available for breakfast, lunch, dinner, or snacks, and complete meals can be purchased in the form of foil-wrapped bars and fortified beverages.

BEST CHOICE: Certified 100% organic products or those produced in a similar or better manner.

CONSIDERATIONS: Some instant foods provide convenience and quality nutrition at the same time; others are less nutritious than their standard counterparts. Comparing labels from each is helpful.

Personal, Psychological & Sociological Aspects:
Basing Choices On How We View Food

Some of the most basic choices in nutrition are tied to our perspectives about food. They often involve considerations other than those related to preferences in taste. Many of our food-related likes, dislikes, and beliefs develop during our early years; others evolve as we age and are usually the result of being confronted with illness or gaining new knowledge about nutrition—or both. These situations frequently result in changes in lifestyle. Eating organic foods, becoming a vegetarian, regulating sugar intake, or following a weight-loss program are common examples. What we eat and how much of it we consume are often based on how foods affect us, or how we perceive they affect us, in terms of health, weight, or energy, or any combination of the three.

When inaccurate, beliefs about food can be difficult to change, even in the face of reason or fact. On the other hand, what we see as an incorrect viewpoint about how a food affects us may actually be accurate for someone else. Since no two people are the same, what applies to one of us simply may not apply to another. The fact that allergies and sensitivities are unique among people is proof of this. We often feel effects from foods, additives, or supplements that are quite different from those experienced by others, including our direct family members.

Ethnicity and religion also impact nutrition. The avoidance of specific foods, beverages, and methods of preparation by various cultures and religious groups is a prime example. Foods that are commonly restricted include beef, eggs, dairy products, pork, fish, and shellfish. In some cases alcohol, coffee, and tea are discouraged or prohibited as well. Beyond restrictions, however, there are often dietary recommendations and requirements. This is evident in the traditional use of unique customary foods and drinks in virtually every culture.

Even our senses evoke thoughts and emotions about particular foods. Food association, in which the sights and smells of foods remind us about people, places, or situations, is built into our thought patterns and affects nutritional choices on a highly individualized basis. Many of our favorite foods became that way not only due to how they taste, but also because of the atmosphere in which they were presented. The same is true of foods we dislike. While we often eat specific foods as a source of comfort when we are anxious, depressed, or ill, the potential also exists for foods to lose their appeal when eaten during times of illness and emotional stress. This is why cancer patients are frequently advised against consuming their favorite foods while undergoing chemotherapy.

Maintaining Our Awareness

Once we learn about the different aspects involved with individual foods and food-related products and have an understanding of how they can affect us, staying alert to new research can help us to maintain our awareness.

The best strategy to accomplish this is to carefully compare current research with past research using the methods outlined in this chapter and then make dietary changes as needed based on our findings. When no past research exists, commentaries from noted experts in the industry are sometimes available and may prove to be helpful.

Chapter 3

*T*he food industry has seen considerable change and development over the past century. Today we use genetic modification to alter the things we eat, hydroponics and aeroponics to grow them, and irradiation to preserve them and protect them from bacteria and parasites. We can, and often do, change their color, texture, flavor, and nutrient content. Our advances include the development of nutraceuticals and food-based supplements as well as a variety of crops that can tolerate herbicides and ward off pests and disease. We have come a long way in terms of food science and technology.

The vast changes the industry has experienced have affected the way foods and related products are produced, processed, packaged, shipped, marketed, priced, stored, prepared, and regulated as well as where and in what form they are consumed. Over the years we have largely replaced home farming with commercial food production, home-cooked meals with fast foods, and basic foods with superfoods. In the process we've manipulated nature and nutrition alike. The result has been a combination of triumphs, difficulties, and uncertainties. Here's a basic look at how each stage of the production-to-consumption chain has been affected:

Production

Pros:
- We now produce more food and can feed more people than at any other point in time.
- Food production is at its fastest.
- We have a greater overall variety of foods and food-related products.
- Instant and easy-to-prepare foods are abundant.
- The development of genetically modified foods is providing greater crop yields and other benefits.
- We have a better awareness of food safety.

- Production-related nutritional technology continues to advance.

Cons:
- Soil erosion due to wind, water, and overuse continues to be a serious global problem that affects the growth and nutritional value of foods.
- A decline in the number of both wild and managed honeybees due to pesticide use and other factors is affecting the pollination of fruits, vegetables, and nuts and may result in serious effects on global food production.[1]
- Fish from various bodies of water have been deemed unsafe for consumption due to industrial pollution.
- Problems related to the use of pesticides, herbicides, fungicides, rodenticides, and microbicides still exist.
- Many animals used for food are being exposed to a variety of chemicals including hormones and antibiotics.
- New, easily preventable diseases have developed among some food animals.
- Hazardous food outbreaks still occur due to improper sanitation and handling.
- Genetically modified foods are being consistently developed and consumed even though their overall and long-term effects on humans and the environment are still unknown.
- The number of foods being produced that are high in fat, salt, sugar, and chemical additives has increased dramatically over the years.
- Genetically modified food plants have been found among standard, non-genetically modified crops.[2]
- Whole foods are often being replaced with refined products that provide little or no fiber, contain chemicals, and have added nutrients in place of those that occur naturally.

---

[1] CCD Steering Committee, "Colony Collapse Disorder Action Plan," USDA, ARS, June 20, 2007, <http://www.ars.usda. gov/is/br/ccd/ccd_actionplan.pdf > (March 22, 2006).
[2] Heald, Paul J. and James Charles Smith, "The Problem of Social Cost in a Genetically Modified Age," 58 Hastings L.J. 87 (2006).

- Government-based regulatory capabilities that are intended to protect the safety and quality of foods cannot keep pace with the industry's growth.

Processing

Pros:
- Foods are processed faster and there are more processing methods than ever before.
- There is a greater range of specialty products available for those who are ill, are unable to digest whole foods, or have dietary restrictions.
- Advances in science have helped establish safer processing procedures to rid foods of harmful bacteria and pathogens including Salmonella and E. coli O157:H7.
- New processing technologies have enhanced the safety, convenience, and palatability of many foods.
- The number of processing methods that effectively destroy pathogens and ward off diseases has increased.
- The number of food products with longer shelf lives and lower spoilage rates has increased.

Cons:
- Certain processing methods, including refining and bleaching, delete naturally occurring nutrients from foods.
- There is greater potential for improper sanitation procedures or machinery errors due to the increased number of food products and manufacturing facilities.
- Processed foods have created the potential for additional food costs. If we buy refined wheat bread, then buy wheat bran and wheat germ to obtain their fiber and nutrients, we have in effect paid three times for the individual parts found in whole wheat.

Shipping

Pros:
- The number of food shipment options has increased.
- Refrigerated shipping is more accessible.
- Foods from all over the world can be easily obtained.
- Out-of-season foods have become readily available through importation from other countries.
- Specialty foods can be acquired more quickly and easily.
- Fast shipping methods allow us to obtain fresher foods and products.

Cons:
- Many foods still lose nutrients during shipping due to heat, light, and time factors.
- The escalating cost of fuel has caused shipping prices, and subsequently food prices, to rise.
- The constant shipment of foods between countries has increased the potential for the transfer of unwanted insects, organisms, and pathogens.
- The percentage of imported foods being inspected is insufficient.

Marketing

Pros:
- The distribution of beneficial information about foods and food-related products has become faster and more widespread.
- Many marketing campaigns have led to trends in healthier eating.
- Consumer exposure to specials and offers for healthful foods and nutritional products has increased.

Cons:
- Deceptive and inaccurate advertising has caused nutritional concerns and health problems for consumers.
- Rising marketing costs have contributed to higher food prices.

- The marketing of foods that are high in fat, salt, sugar, and/or chemical additives has increased.
- The number of ads that encourage overeating has increased.

Packaging & Storage

Pros:
- There is a greater amount of information and education about food storage safety.
- Many foods can be stored for longer periods of time due to advances in production and packaging.
- There is a wider variety of food packaging and storage materials.
- Refrigeration is more convenient and accessible.

Cons:
- Despite advances in food storage safety and consumer education, there are still millions of cases of foodborne illness each year, hundreds of which result in death.[3]
- The storage of food in improper containers continues to pose health risks.
- A greater number of packaging materials contain chemicals that have the potential to leach into foods.

Preparation

Pros:
- We now know a great deal about food preparation safety.
- There are more food preparation techniques and tools than ever before.

---

[3] Mead, Paul S., et al., "Food-Related Illness and Death in the United States," *Emerging Infectious Diseases, Volume 5, No. 5,* September-October 1999, <http://www.cdc.gov/ ncidod/eid/vol5no5/mead.htm> (March 27, 2007).

65

- Proper preparation has helped to ward off disease and provide a higher level of nutrition.
- The development of different preparation styles has provided variety in the diet.

Cons:
- The preparation of food in improper containers (including those that contain lead or other toxic materials that can leach into foods) continues to pose health risks.
- Unsanitary food preparation conditions and improper preparation procedures still result in serious illnesses and deaths each year.

Consumption

Pros:
- Education about nutrition and food safety has increased substantially.
- Food-related diseases are more readily preventable and treatable.
- Foods can be obtained more conveniently, day or night.
- Healthy foods that are low in fat, salt, and sugar and contain no chemical additives are abundant and easily accessible.
- New technology and improved strategies allow us to control hazardous food outbreaks with greater speed and precision.

Cons:
- The number of foods being consumed that are high in fat, salt, sugar, and/or chemical additives has increased dramatically over the years.
- The prevalence of overweight and obesity among children, adolescents, and adults continues to be a serious health concern.
- The incidence of gastrointestinal problems, many of which are due to overeating or other poor eating habits, is at an all-time high.[4]

---

[4] National Institutes of Health, National Digestive Diseases Information Clearinghouse, "Digestive Diseases Statistics," *NIH Publication No. 06–3873,* December 2005, <http://digestive.niddk.nih.gov/statistics/statistics.htm> (December 8, 2007).

- The system designed to allow us to control hazardous food outbreaks with greater speed and precision still needs improvement.

More On Marketing

Much of the influence marketing has on nutrition is driven by intense competition for food product sales. This influence can be good or bad, depending on the quality and nutritional value of advertised products, the accuracy and usefulness of product ads and labels, and other factors. Unfortunately, some ads and labels are misleading. For example, one magazine ad for a popular powdered drink mix has pictures of fruit in it, when in actuality there is no fruit whatsoever in the product, a fact disclosed in fine print at the bottom of the page. The problem is most of us don't have the time or inclination to read the fine print, and are likely to think that what we see is what's in the product. The ad's main wording further directly implies that the product is healthy, when in fact it contains several chemicals and is of questionable nutritional value.

In addition to these types of marketing tactics, persuasive advertising and marketing catch phrases known as "calls to action" are constantly used to get us to purchase products. "Buy some today," "Try it soon," "Don't wait to get some," and "Hurry and try them" are just a few examples.

Sales are also promoted through repetitive consumer exposure to food product advertising. Food company marketers utilize a number of avenues to gain that exposure, including through ads on the radio, television, and internet; in newspapers and newsletters; on billboards; and at the movies, and more recently by having celebrities and sports figures visibly use brand name products during televised programs and events. Companies also use signs, posters, coupons, contests, and giveaways. Clever names, catchy tunes, and the use of words such as health, healthy, natural, nature, whole, and wholesome are often used to push products that offer little in the way of nutrition and may actually cause nutritional deficits.

A host of tactics are also used to make foods look bigger and more attractive, and therefore more marketable. Oranges often have artificially colored skins; walnuts often have artificially colored shells. Butter and cheeses are frequently tinted with beta carotene (an antioxidant and also a precursor to vitamin A found in orange and yellow fruits and vegetables) or annatto (a dye obtained from the seeds of the annatto tree) to give them a yellow or orange hue. Many farm-raised salmon are fed color-enhancement pellets to produce filets that are bright coral in color.

Still another method of promoting food product sales, and more commonly the sale of dietary supplements, is the use of strong endorsements from doctors, attorneys, or others of notable standing. In many cases, however, these individuals have vested financial interests in the product or product line being promoted. The FDA requires the following statement to be printed on food product and dietary supplement labels as well as on all related marketing materials in which claims about food products or dietary supplements are made: "This statement has not been evaluated by the FDA. This product is not intended to diagnose, treat, cure, or prevent any disease."

From a commercial angle, restaurant and food service company advertising often attempts to lure us with specials, pictures of appetizing foods and beverages, variety, convenient locations, and even the type of atmosphere they offer. Unfortunately many featured foods and beverages are high in fat, salt, or sugar, or any combination of the three, though a growing number of establishments are now offering and advertising healthier alternatives.

Marketing to Children

Advertising and marketing geared toward children and teens also has a major impact on nutrition. Many food-related television commercials aired between cartoons and other children's programs are not focused on promoting health, but rather are designed to play on children's emotions and self-esteem in an effort to increase sales. Children are often given the idea that in order to be important, cool, respected, cute, attractive, funny, energetic, athletic, or possess some other critical trait—including good health—they need to eat a certain food or drink a certain beverage, whether that food or beverage in itself is a healthy choice or not. Some ads feature favorite cartoon characters, though there are also numerous others that feature athletes, musicians, and actors who kids relate to, look up to, and are prone to emulate the behaviors of, especially in front of other kids. These ads not only appear on television; they are also at the movies, on the radio, in magazines, on the internet, and on posters. There are also contests and giveaways. For many kids, drinking or eating what the icons eat or drink, what the icons *say* they eat or drink, or what the icons *appear* to eat or drink in the ads is a form of identity, a way to get attention and recognition. Others believe their abilities will be enhanced simply by eating or drinking the featured foods or beverages. As a result, actual individual preferences or considerations of what's healthy may have little to do with the choices a child makes when selecting foods and beverages. For example, many kids are affected by "pour pressure," a phenomenon in which they feel compelled to drink sodas and other high-sugar, low-nutrient drinks on a regular basis due to the fact that their friends are drinking them, even at school. Fortunately, a number of school boards across the nation have recognized the potential for health problems from excessive consumption of soft drinks and have pulled them from school vending machines, stores, and snack bars.

Overall, the promotion of poor eating habits geared toward children via advertising helps set the stage for disease early in life. When an animated character pops on a television screen and kicks an apple to promote the idea that a sugar-filled, artificially flavored, artificially colored, preservative-filled, nutrient-lacking, fiberless snack tastes better, the message that comes across is one of overall preference based solely on taste, and it teaches children that whole foods have less value than other less nutritious foods. Since children are impressionable and learn by example, giving them any reason to avoid fruits or vegetables filled with fiber, vitamins, minerals, antioxidants, and enzymes and promoting them to prefer foods with empty calories or little nutritional value instead simply isn't a good idea. Mocking sound nutrition is a devious way to gain profits, plain and simple.

The Federal Trade Commission (FTC) is responsible for the regulation of food advertising. The Food Marketing Institute, an entity that deals with food handling issues, also plays a role.

Federal Trade Commission (FTC)
Consumer Response Center
CRC-240
Washington, DC 20580
877-FTC-HELP (877-382-4357)
www.ftc.gov

Food Marketing Institute
2345 Crystal Drive
Suite 800
Arlington, VA 22202
202.452.8444
www.fmi.org

Regulatory Effects On Nutrition

Regulation of the industry is another area that affects consumer nutrition. While it is intended to help ensure the safety, quality, sanitary production, and accurate representation of foods and food-related products, there are a number of political and economic factors that often impede on its goals—and ultimately affect consumers. Among them, business interests and lobbying power have the strongest influence, often causing legislative, legal, regulatory, and public policy issues to impede on nutrition and the sciences that back it. The result is less focus on scientific fact, which gets lost in the traffic somewhere between profits and power. The magnitude of the situation is far-reaching. These issues not only cause confusion and frustration for the consumer, but also for those who regulate the industry and work in it. The following summarized statements and portions of statements compiled during a public workshop held by the Committee to Ensure Safe Food From Production to Consumption express the industry's views on the importance of utilizing science in maintaining and improving our food supply:[5]

"The separation of regulatory efforts from research efforts is likely to lead to better science."

"...supports HACCP, partnerships, and the use of science and technology..."

"...farmers want to produce safe food based on sound science (not headlines)."

"...agencies need resources: scientists and dollars."

"...resist knee-jerk reactions, show leadership, less political science, and more real science..."

"...shifting to science-based, preventive framework is the right track..."

"...agencies need to be open-minded, science based..."

"...need science based information to make decisions..."

"...media has great power..."

Nutrition-related problems also tend to occur when regulatory requirements are ignored or improperly followed, and when unforeseen circumstances arise due to the use of new food technologies. Other areas for potential issues include those in which foods (both foreign and domestic) carry regulatory exemptions.

---

[5] Institute of Medicine, National Research Council. Ensuring Safe Food From Production to Consumption, pp. 169-177. Washington, D.C. Reprinted with permission from the National Academies Press. Copyright © 1998 National Academy of Sciences.

Industry regulation is both internal and external. Self-regulation is carried out internally by corporations, groups, associations, tribes, and other entities, while external regulation is performed by the government. Regulatory programs, systems, and efforts exist at international, national, regional, state, and local levels. In the U.S. the four main government agencies responsible for overseeing federal food regulations are the U.S. Food and Drug Administration (FDA), the U.S. Department of Agriculture (USDA) Food Safety and Inspection Service (FSIS), the Environmental Protection Agency (EPA), and NOAA's National Marine Fisheries Service (NMFS). Here's a closer look at each of them and what they do:

1. The U.S. Food & Drug Administration (FDA)

The FDA is part of the Department of Health and Human Services (DHHS). Through its Center for Food Safety & Applied Nutrition (CFSAN) it oversees the production, processing, packaging, and storage of domestic and imported foods (except those that fall under the jurisdiction of the USDA), as well as detainment of such foods when necessary.

The FDA's CFSAN regulates:

- the safety and labeling of bottled water.

- the safety and labeling of wine and wine beverages with less than 7 percent alcohol content (the Alcohol & Tobacco Tax and Trade Bureau regulates those with an alcohol content of 7 percent or greater).

- the labeling of foods other than those solely regulated by the USDA, to ensure that they are accurate and informative.

- the safety of all foods except traditional, non-game meat and poultry (FDA *does* regulate game meats, such as venison and snake). This includes medical foods and infant formulas, and foods (including animal feed) derived from genetically modified (also referred to as "bioengineered," "biotech," or "genetically engineered") crops.

* the safety of all ingredients used in food products. The FDA is also responsible for approving new food additives.

* the safety of dietary supplements.

* pesticides (this is a three-way effort performed together with the USDA and the EPA; the FDA and the USDA are specifically responsible for monitoring pesticide residues in the products they regulate to ensure they do not exceed allowable levels).

* drug residues in milk, eggs, and meat (this is a dual effort together with the USDA).

In addition, the FDA promotes the use of Hazard Analysis Critical Control Point (HACCP) programs, an effective and highly utilized food safety monitoring system that was initially used by NASA and is based on the prevention of hazardous situations that can lead to foodborne illness.

U. S. Food and Drug Administration (FDA)
5600 Fishers Lane
Rockville, MD 20857-0001
1-888-INFO-FDA (1-888-463-6332)
www.fda.gov

U.S. Food and Drug Administration
Center For Food Safety & Applied Nutrition (CFSAN)
5100 Paint Branch Parkway
College Park, MD 20740-3835
1-888-INFO-FDA (1-888-463-6332)
www.cfsan.fda.gov

U.S. Food and Drug Administration/University of Maryland
Joint Institute For Food Safety & Applied Nutrition
1122 Patapsco Building
University of Maryland
College Park, MD 20740
301-314-6806
www.FoodRisk.org

National Center for Food Safety & Technology (NCFST)
6502 South Archer Road
Summit-Argo, IL 60501
708-563-1576
Contact: Britt Burton Freeman, Ph.D.

2. The United States Department of Agriculture's (USDA's) Food Safety and Inspection Service (FSIS)

Established in 1862 by President Abraham Lincoln, the USDA is the oldest federal food-monitoring agency. Through its Food Safety and Inspection Service (FSIS) it oversees the safety, wholesomeness, accurate labeling, and proper packaging of foreign and domestic meat, poultry, and egg products (the FDA regulates shell eggs). It is also responsible for the regulation of herbicide-tolerant crops. The USDA works closely with the FDA and the Environmental Protection Agency (EPA).

USDA Meat & Poultry Hotline
The Hotline answers consumer food safety questions and provides support for food safety educators and communicators.

Meat & Poultry Hotline:
1-888-MPHotline (1-888-674-6854)
1-800-256-7072 (TTY)

3. The Environmental Protection Agency (EPA)
The Office of Prevention, Pesticides, and Toxic Substances

Established in July 1970, the EPA sets maximum allowable levels for pesticide residues in or on food, including animal feed. The agency also works to protect the food supply from chemical and microbial contamination, promotes the use of safer forms of pest control, and develops national standards for drinking water obtained from public water systems.

The EPA regulates:

- tap water from municipal water sources, schools, businesses, homeowner associations, campgrounds, and shopping malls.

- the sale and use of pesticides, including those in the form of biotechnology used to develop pest-resistant plants. The testing of foods to determine if pesticide levels exceed allowable amounts, however, is performed by the FDA and USDA. If elevated levels are found, the FDA is responsible for taking corrective action.

U.S. Environmental Protection Agency
Ariel Rios Building
1200 Pennsylvania Avenue, N.W.
Washington, D.C. 20460
202-564-7864
www.epa.gov

4. NOAA National Marine Fisheries Service (NMFS)

NOAA's National Marine Fisheries Service (NMFS) is a division of the Department of Commerce. Its mission includes monitoring seafood for health and safety. It maintains several laboratories dedicated to achieving this mission, where marine animals, ocean water, and sediment are tested for a wide range of issues including bacteria and contaminants. The NMFS has authority to close fisheries and fishing grounds during environmental incidents that cause seafood to be unsafe, such as red tide.

NOAA National Marine Fisheries Service
Office of Public Affairs
1315 East West Highway, 14th Floor
Silver Spring, MD 20910
301-713-2370 / www.nmfs.noaa.gov

Each of these federal regulatory agencies collaborates with other assisting federal agencies (some of which play less prominent regulatory roles), as well as with state and local governments, foreign liaisons, professional organizations, universities, private businesses, and individuals.

Other Assisting Federal Agencies

The USDA's Center for Nutrition Policy and Promotion (CNPP)

Established in 1994 as part of USDA's Food, Nutrition, and Consumer Services (FNCS), the Center for Nutrition Policy and Promotion (CNPP) conducts applied research and analyses in nutrition and consumer economics. The Center also works to advance and promote dietary guidance for consumers, such as through the development of the MyPyramid Food Guidance System released in April of 2005 (which replaced the original Food Guide Pyramid of 1992).

Center for Nutrition Policy and Promotion
3101 Park Center Drive, 10th Floor
Alexandria, VA 22302-1594
703-305-7600
703-305-3300 fax
www.cnpp.usda.gov

The USDA's Food and Nutrition Service (FNS)

This division of the USDA's Food, Nutrition, and Consumer Services administers the USDA's nutrition assistance programs. The FNS works together with cooperating organizations to increase food security and reduce hunger by providing children and low-income people access to food, a healthy diet, and nutrition education. Programs associated with the FNS include the Food Stamp Program, WIC (Women, Infants, and Children), and the National School Lunch Program.

Food & Nutrition Service
3101 Park Center Drive
Alexandria, VA 22302
www.fns.usda.gov

The USDA's Agricultural Marketing Service (AMS)

The AMS performs a number of different functions through a variety of commodity programs, including overseeing marketing agreements and orders, administering research and promotion programs, and purchasing commodities for Federal food programs. Although not a major federal regulatory agency, the AMS does enforce some federal laws, including the Perishable Agricultural Commodities Act and the Federal Seed Act. Through its Science and Technology Program it also oversees the USDA's Pesticide Data Program (PDP), which tests for pesticide residues in foods and beverages, including finished drinking water. The AMS is also in charge of the USDA National Organic Program (NOP).

Agricultural Marketing Service
Office of Public Affairs
1400 Independence Avenue, S.W.
Washington, D.C. 20250
202.720.8998
www.ams.usda.gov

USDA National Organic Program
1400 Independence Avenue, S.W., Room 2632-S
Washington, DC 20250
202.720.8998
www.usda.gov/nop

The USDA's Animal & Plant Health Inspection Service (APHIS)

Among its many functions, the USDA's Animal and Plant Health Inspection Service (APHIS), through its Biotechnology Regulatory Services division, regulates genetically engineered or "biotech" crops to ensure that they do not pose a risk to plant or animal health. APHIS is also responsible for approving and licensing biotech substances for veterinary use, including animal vaccines.

Animal and Plant Health Inspection Service
1400 Independence Avenue, S.W.
Washington, D.C. 20250
www.aphis.usda.gov

The USDA's Grain Inspection, Packers, and Stockyards Administration (GIPSA)

The Grain Inspection, Packers and Stockyards Administration (GIPSA) facilitates the marketing of livestock, poultry, meat, cereals, oilseeds, and related agricultural products, and promotes fair and competitive trading practices for the overall benefit of consumers and American agriculture.

GIPSA Administrator
Stop 3601, Room 2055-South Building
1400 Independence Avenue, S.W.
Washington, D.C. 20250-3601
202-720-0219 / www.gipsa.usda.gov

The USDA's Agricultural Research Service (ARS)

The Agricultural Research Service (ARS) is the USDA's chief scientific research agency. Its focus is to develop and implement solutions to agricultural problems that affect food and nutrition (especially those of high national priority), assess the nutritional needs of Americans, and continually ensure safe, high-quality foods and agricultural products. The ARS oversees 1200 research projects within 22 national programs with the assistance of 2100 scientists in 100 research locations.

Agricultural Research Service
Jamie L. Whitten Building
Room 302A
1400 Independence Avenue, S.W.
Washington, D.C. 20250
202-720-3656
202-720-5427 fax
www.ars.usda.gov

The USDA's Cooperative State Research, Education, and Extension Service (CSREES)

Through its Food, Nutrition & Health programs the CSREES strengthens the nation's ability to address issues related to diet, health, food safety, food security, and food science and technology.

Cooperative State Research, Education, and Extension Service
1400 Independence Avenue S.W.
Stop 2201
Washington, D.C. 20250-2201
202-720-7441
www.csrees.usda.gov

The USDA's Economic Research Service (ERS)

ERS research examines the effect of economic factors (including prices, income, and demographics), nutrition education, and food policy on food choices and dietary quality. From a food safety perspective, ERS research is designed and utilized to enhance the efficiency and effectiveness of public food safety policies and programs. ERS food safety research focuses on analyzing the costs of human illness due to foodborne disease and assessing food safety incentives and activities of industry, consumers, and government.

Economic Research Service
1800 M Street, N.W.
Washington, D.C. 20036-5831
202-694-5050 (8 a.m. to 5 p.m. E.S.T., Monday-Friday)
www.ers.usda.gov

The USDA's Codex Alimentarius Commission

The Codex Alimentarius Commission is a major international liaison that encourages fair international food trade while promoting the health and economic interest of consumers. The Commission's U.S. contact point is the U.S. Codex Office, a branch of the USDA's Food Safety and Inspection Service (FSIS). The Codex Office staff work closely with the U.S. delegates to various committees, as well as government agencies, members of Congress, non-governmental agencies and members of the general public.

Codex Alimentarius Commission
South Building, Room 4861
1400 Independence Avenue, S.W.
Washington, D.C. 20250
202-205-7760
202-720-3157 fax
email: uscodex@fsis.usda.gov

Centers for Disease Control and Prevention (CDC)

Established in 1946, this division of the U.S. Department of Health and Human Services investigates food-related illnesses and keeps tabs on the number of outbreaks. It also provides assistance to state and local agencies (such as health departments) when they request it, and distributes information about foodborne illness prevention. The CDC works closely with the FDA, EPA, and USDA.

Centers for Disease Control and Prevention
1600 Clifton Road, Atlanta, GA 30333
800-CDC-INFO (800-232-4636)
www.cdc.gov

National Institutes of Health (NIH)

Part of the Department of Health and Human Services, the NIH indirectly yet substantially assists in promoting both new and continued research on food-related pathogens and in providing direction as to which areas of public health and disease—including those related to nutrition—can benefit from intervention. The NIH provides additional useful information through its National Toxicology Program by producing a biennial Report on Carcinogens that identifies and discusses agents, substances, mixtures, or circumstances of exposure, including those associated with food, that have the potential to pose a human health hazard due to their carcinogenicity. The NIH also collaborates with the National Library of Medicine to offer MedlinePlus, a health information service that provides a variety of food, nutrition, and food safety topics.

National Institutes of Health
9000 Rockville Pike
Bethesda, Maryland 20892
301-496-4000 / 301-402-9612 (TTY)
www.nih.gov

81

The Alcohol and Tobacco Tax and Trade Bureau

Part of the U.S. Treasury Department, the Alcohol and Tobacco Tax and Trade Bureau regulates the labeling and quality of most alcoholic beverages (wine and wine beverages with less than 7% alcohol content are regulated by the FDA).

Alcohol and Tobacco Tax and Trade Bureau
Public Information Officer
1310 G Street, N.W., Suite 300
Washington, D.C. 20220
202-927-5000
www.ttb.treas.gov
email: ttbquestions@ttb.treas.gov

U.S. Customs and Border Protection

A division of the U.S. Department of Homeland Security, U.S. Customs and Border Protection has the responsibility and authority to check and detain foods and related imports as necessary according to federal guidelines.

U.S. Customs and Border Protection
1300 Pennsylvania Avenue, N.W.
Washington, D.C. 20229
877-CBP-5511 (877-227-5511)
www.cbp.gov

An excellent overview regarding federal regulation of the food industry can be viewed online at http://edis.ifas.ufl.edu/FS121.

International Assistance

In addition to the international efforts set forth by the USDA's Codex Alimentarius Commission and other U.S. agencies, there are a number of foreign international agencies that also collaborate on global nutritional issues. They include:

- The World Health Organization (WHO)
- The Food and Agriculture Organization (FAO)
- The European Food Safety Authority (EFSA)
- The World Food Safety Organization (WFSO)

Among these, the United Nations' World Health Organization (WHO), with membership of 193 countries and two associate members,[6] has the broadest influence on addressing nutrition-related health issues at a global level. Although not a regulatory agency, WHO works closely with the United Nations' Food and Agriculture Organization (FAO) and Department of Food Safety, Zoonoses, and Foodborne Diseases (FOS), as well as with other agencies and organizations, its members, and the private sector to set policies, promote research, and help countries address public health issues. WHO is an important vehicle in achieving food safety and security and in providing a united system for effectively improving nutrition-related healthcare worldwide.

World Health Organization
Avenue Appia 20
CH - 1211 Geneva 27
Switzerland
+41 22 791 2111
+41 22 791 3111 fax

---

[6] World Health Organization, "Working for health: an introduction to the World Health Organization," June 20, 2007, <http://www.who.int/about/brochure_en.pdf> (December 8, 2007).

83

Other Regulatory Support

There are also a number of consumer groups, professional organizations, trade associations, and universities that either support government regulatory efforts or promote the development of better regulations, or both. These entities assist through programs, training, continued education, funding, research, and other avenues, and in many cases collaborate with federal regulatory agencies on nutritional issues. Those that represent consumers include the following:

- **The Center For Science In The Public Interest (CSPI)**
  1875 Connecticut Avenue, N.W., Suite 300
  Washington, D.C. 20009
  202-332-9110
  www.cspinet.org

- **Consumer's Union**
  101 Truman Avenue
  Yonkers, NY 10703-1057
  914-378-2000
  www.consumerreports.org

- **The Center for Food Safety**
  660 Pennsylvania Avenue, S.E., Suite 302
  Washington, D.C. 20003
  www.centerforfoodsafety.org

- **The Consumer Federation of America**
  1620 I Street, S.W., Suite 200
  Washington, D.C. 20006
  202-387-6121
  www.consumerfed.org

- **The National Consumers League**
  1701 K Street, N.W., Suite 1200
  Washington, D.C. 20006
  202-835-3323 / 202-835-0747 fax
  www.nclnet.org

- **Safe Tables Our Priority**
  3149 Dundee Road, Suite 276
  Northbrook, IL 60062
  847-831-3032 phone/fax
  www.safetables.org

Chapter 4

*W*hether by habit, preference, or a combination of the two, many of us consume a diet that consistently contains the same foods. If that diet consists of a variety of complex carbohydrates (fruits, vegetables, grains, and legumes), along with a lesser proportion of low-fat dairy products, lean meats, and healthy seafood (with adaptations if we're vegetarian or have dietary restrictions), our likelihood of achieving and maintaining better health is increased. If not, we're more likely to run into nutrition-related health problems sooner or later.

Often we routinely eat the foods we eat simply because they taste good and are convenient to obtain, without realizing the short- or long-term effects they can have on our bodies. Learning about their nutritional value and the effects they can have, however, can help us to make better dietary choices. Complex carbohydrates, for example, are beneficial because they provide fiber, vitamins, minerals, and antioxidants, are low in fat, and are cholesterol free. Some, including beans, peas, and whole grain rice, even provide protein. Dairy products, meats, fish, and seafood provide protein, fats, and other nutrients. All of these foods provide our bodies with the essentials they need for efficient functioning and rebuilding. When the foods we consume are organic, we also lessen our potential exposure to synthetic pesticides, fertilizers, and other chemicals.

In deciphering whether a food or beverage is one that we should consume or avoid, or consume less or more of, comparing its probable or proven effects—both positive and negative—can help steer us in the right direction. Provided here are some of the pros and cons associated with many of the more commonly consumed foods and beverages:

1. Bread

Pros:
- Provides carbohydrates, protein, and other nutrients, along with varying amounts of fiber.
- Is produced from a variety of grains.
- Whole grain versions provide complex carbohydrates, good amounts of fiber, and a wide variety of naturally occurring (rather than manually added) vitamins, minerals, and other nutrients.
- Consuming fiber in whole grain breads reduces the risk of coronary heart disease, may help prevent constipation and hemorrhoids, and may help with weight management.[1]
- Many breads are cholesterol free, fat free, or both.
- Some breads contain added beneficial fiber.
- Consuming breads fortified with folate before and during pregnancy helps prevent neural tube defects during fetal development.

Cons:
- Many breads are made with bleached and bromated refined grains, which are lower in fiber and naturally occurring nutrients than whole grains (some nutrients, though generally not all, are added back after refinement).
- Many breads provide no fiber at all.
- Many breads contain artificial colors, flavors, and preservatives and other chemical additives.
- Some breads are high in sugar.
- Brown bread is not necessarily whole grain bread.
- Breads made with gluten-containing grains (namely wheat, barley, and rye) need to be avoided by those with celiac disease or gluten sensitivity.
- Conventionally produced breads and bread products may contain residues from applied pesticides, herbicides, fungicides, rodenticides, or other chemicals (or a combination of these).

---

[1] United States Department of Agriculture, "Grains," *MyPyramid.gov.,* September 11, 2008, <http://www.mypyramid.gov/pyramid/grains_why_print.html> December 2, 2008.

2. Beef

Pros:
- High in protein.
- A source of complete protein, containing all nine essential amino acids.
- A good source of zinc, iron, niacin, and B vitamins (riboflavin, niacin, thiamin, B_6, and B_{12}).
- Many cuts are lean.
- About half the fatty acids found in beef are monounsaturated, the same type found in olive, canola, and peanut oils.[2]
- Irradiated meats may be useful in preventing foodborne illnesses, especially among those with compromised immune systems.
- Beef is a source of conjugated linoleic acid (CLA), a trans fatty acid and naturally occurring anticarcinogen (cancer-fighting agent) that may have health benefits.[3,4,5]

Cons:
- Beef that is not organic may contain residues of antibiotics, hormones, pesticides, or other chemicals.
- Many cuts have a high fat content.
- Low in fiber.
- Low in nutrients other than zinc, iron, niacin, and B vitamins (riboflavin, niacin, thiamin, B_6, and B_{12}).
- May be treated with coloring agents and preservatives.

---

[2] Whetsell, M.S., Rayburn, E.B., and Lozier, J.D., "Human Health Effects of Fatty Acids in Beef," West Virginia University Extension Service, *Pasture-based Beef Systems for Appalachia,* August 2003, <http://www.wvu.edu/ ~agexten/forglvst/humanhealth.pdf> March 9, 2009.

[3] Mir, P. S., et al., "Conjugated linoleic acid-enriched beef production," *American Journal of Clinical Nutrition,* Vol. 79, No. 6, 1207S-1211S, June 2004, <http://www.ajcn.org/cgi/content/abstract/79/6/1207S>. December 2, 2008.

[4] Gaullier, J.M., et al., "Conjugated linoleic acid supplementation for 1 y reduced body fat mass in healthy overweight humans," *American Journal of Clinical Nutrition,* Vol. 79, No. 6, 1118-25, June 2004, <http://www.ajcn.org/cgi/content/abstract/79/6/1118>. December 2, 2008.

[5] Kelly, M.L., et al., "Dietary fatty acid sources affect conjugated linoleic acid concentrations in milk from lactating dairy cows," *Journal of Nutrition,* May 1998; 128(5): 881-5.

- May be exposed to a mix of gases, including carbon monoxide, to maintain its color, potentially allowing spoiled or near spoiled meat to appear fresh.[6]
- Beef that is not cooked thoroughly until done to destroy any potential foodborne organisms may cause illness.
- Overcooked beef (as well as other meats) may present a cancer hazard due to the production of chemicals called heterocyclic amines.[7]
- Smoked beef or beef that has had smoke flavoring added may contain carcinogenic (cancer-causing) chemicals.[8] This is also true of other meats and fish that have undergone the same treatment.
- Beef, like other meats and meat products, can carry harmful bacteria that cannot be seen or smelled, including Salmonella, Campylobacter jejuni, Escherichia coli O157:H7, Listeria monocytogenes, Clostridium perfringens, and Staphylococcus aureus.
- Beef can carry various parasites, though they can be destroyed by thorough cooking.

3. Pork

Pros:
- High in protein.
- A source of complete protein, containing all nine essential amino acids.
- Many cuts, including pork tenderloin, are lean.
- Contains several B vitamins.
- Contains numerous minerals, including calcium, potassium, and iron.

---

[6] Copyright © 2006 by Consumers Union of U.S., Inc. Yonkers, NY 10703-1057, a nonprofit organization. Reprinted with permission from the July 2006 issue of CONSUMER REPORTS® for educational purposes only. No commercial use or reproduction permitted. For more information visit: www.ConsumerReports.org; www.GreenerChoices.org; www.eco-labels.org.

[7] U.S. Dept. of Health and Human Services, Public Health Service, National Toxicology Program, "Report on Carcinogens," 11th Edition, December 2004.

[8] Gomaa, E.A., et al., "Polycyclic aromatic hydrocarbons in smoked food products and commercial liquid smoke flavourings," *Food Additives & Contaminants,* September-October 1993; 10(5): 503-21. Taylor & Francis Ltd. <http://www.informaworld.com> Reprinted by permission of the publisher.

- By law, no hormones are allowed to be administered to hogs used for consumption.

Cons:
- Low in fiber.
- Some cuts have a high fat content.
- Antibiotics are allowed to be administered to hogs used for food, creating a risk—although small—that antibiotic residues may be found in some pork.
- Most conventionally produced ham and bacon has been smoked or contains smoke flavoring, two situations that can cause the meat to have carcinogens, and which in turn may cause negative effects on health.[9]
- Pork that is not cooked thoroughly until done to destroy any potential foodborne organisms may cause illness.
- Overcooked pork may present a cancer hazard.[10]
- Pork, like other meats and meat products, can carry harmful bacteria that cannot be seen or smelled, including Salmonella, Escherichia coli O157:H7, Campylobacter jejuni, Listeria monocytogenes, Clostridium perfringens, and Staphylococcus aureus.
- Pork can carry parasites, particularly Toxoplasma gondii, though they can be destroyed by thorough cooking.[11]

4. Seafood (Fish & Shellfish)

Pros:
- High in protein.
- Good source of B vitamins.

---

[9] Anderson, J., "Nutrition and Cancer: Quick Facts," Colorado State University Extension, *Publication 9.313,* August 2008, <http://www.ext.colostate.edu/Pubs/foodnut/09313.html>.

[10] U.S. Dept. of Health and Human Services, Public Health Service, National Toxicology Program, *Report on Carcinogens,* 11th Edition, December 2004.

[11] Satin, Morton. Food Alert!: The Ultimate Sourcebook for Food Safety, p. 236. New York: Checkmark Books. Copyright © 1999.

- Good source of minerals, including iron.
- Low in fat.
- Fish, especially salmon and sardines, are an excellent source of omega fatty acids.
- Canned fish with soft bones (e.g., sardines, anchovies, and salmon) is a good source of calcium.
- Some fish, including salmon, catfish, and freshwater trout, do not contain high levels of mercury.
- Mollusks, such as clams, oysters, scallops, and mussels, have been found to contain a large percentage of noncholesterol sterols that inhibit the absorption of cholesterol eaten at the same meal.[12]

Cons:
- Both fish and crustacean shellfish (shrimp, crab, lobster, etc.) are common allergens.
- Some types of fish, including shark, swordfish, tilefish, king mackerel, and some species of fresh, frozen, and canned tuna, are high in mercury. Canned white albacore tuna is higher in mercury content than canned light tuna.
- Many types of seafood sold commercially are treated with chemical additives including phosphates and sulfites, which may cause health issues.
- Seafood may be treated with carbon monoxide or filtered smoke gas to maintain or enhance its color. This is a common practice with tuna used as sushi.
- Salmon, particularly that which is farmed, often carries organochlorine contaminants including dioxins and PCBs (polychlorinated biphenyls), which are reasonably anticipated to be human carcinogens.[13,14] Removing the skin can reduce the amount of contaminants.

---

[12] Delaware Sea Grant College Program, "Seafood Nutritional Information," *Cholesterol,* n.d., <http://www.ocean.udel.edu/seagrant/outreach/seafood/nutritioninfo.html> December 2008.
[13] World Health Organization, "PCBs and dioxins in salmon," June 20, 2007, <http://www.who.int/foodsafety/chem/pcbsalmon/en/index.html> December 8, 2007.
[14] U.S. Department of Health and Human Services, Public Health Service, National Toxicology Program, "Polychlorinated Biphenyls (PCBs)," *Report on Carcinogens,* 11th Edition, December 2004,

- Seafood and seafood products can carry harmful bacteria that cannot be seen or detected by smell, including Salmonella, E. coli, Clostridium botulinum, Clostridium perfringens, Lysteria monocytogenes, Vibrio (including Vibrio cholerae, Vibrio fulnificus, and other Vibrio species), Yersinia enterocolitica, Shigella, and Staphylococcus aureus.
- Seafood can carry parasites, though they can be destroyed by thorough cooking or freezing.[15]
- Seafood can carry viruses (including the Norwalk Virus) that cause gastrointestinal illness.
- Seafood can carry poisonous toxins that cause Ciguatera, Tetrodotoxin, Scombroid, or Shellfish poisoning.
- Seafood may be exposed to sewage, industrial waste, or agricultural run-off (or any combination of these); may carry toxins, bacteria, or viruses; and may contain residual chemicals including pesticides, additives, and antibiotics (or other drugs).[16] While this is true of both wild-caught and farmed seafood, incidence is likely to be higher with that which is farmed.
- Although often considered a delicacy, the green gland in American lobsters (also called Maine lobsters) known as the tomalley is likely to contain contaminants that cause Paralytic Shellfish Poisoning. To view the July 2008 advisory on this topic go to **http://www.fda.gov/bbs/topics /NEWS/2008/NEW 01866.html**.

5. Chicken

Pros:
- High in protein.

<http://ntp.niehs.nih.gov/ ntp/roc/eleventh/profiles/s149pcb.pdf> December 3, 2008.

[15] United States Food and Drug Administration, CFSAN, "The Safe Food Chart," *Meat, Poultry, and Seafood*, 2007, <http://www.cfsan.fda.gov/~dms/fttmeat.html> December 3, 2008.

[16] U.S. Department of Agriculture, APHIS, CEI, "Outbreak of Shrimp Viral Disease in Central America: Situation Report," June 1999, <http://www.aphis.usda.gov/vs/ceah/cei/taf/emergingdieasenotice_files/ shrimp.htm> December 3, 2008.

- Fresh roasted skinless chicken breast provides B vitamins, potassium, calcium, iron, vitamin A, and vitamin C.
- White meat (breast and wing meat) is lower in fat.
- No hormones are allowed to be administered to chickens that are used for consumption.

Cons:

- May contain residues of antibiotics, pesticides, arsenic, or other chemical additives.
- Dark meat and skin are high in fat.
- Chicken products, including whole packaged chickens and chicken parts, often contain high-sodium broth or have been treated with a solution that is high in sodium. They also often contain chemical additives.
- Chicken, like other meats and meat products, can carry harmful bacteria that cannot be seen or detected by smell, including Salmonella, Escherichia coli O157:H7, Campylobacter jejuni, Listeria monocytogenes, Clostridium perfringens, and Staphylococcus aureus.
- Chicken can carry parasites, though they can be destroyed by thorough cooking.

6. Chocolate

Pros:

- May create pleasurable feelings or enhance mood by affecting human brain chemistry.[17]
- Is unlikely to be a cause of acne.[18]
- Both milk and dark chocolate have antioxidants, though dark chocolate (particularly in the form of natural cocoa powder) has naturally higher antioxidant value (approximately double that of milk chocolate).[19]

---

[17] Kuwana, Ellen, "Discovering the Sweet Mysteries of Chocolate," *Neuroscience For Kids,* n.d., <http://faculty.washington.edu/chudler/choco.html> December 4, 2008.
[18] National Institutes of Health, NIAMS, "Acne," January 2006, <http://www.niams.nih.gov/Health_Info/Acne/#acne_c> March 8, 2009.
[19] Ding, E.L., et al., "Chocolate and Prevention of Cardiovascular Disease: A Systematic Review," *Nutrition & Metabolism,* 2006, 3:2, <http://nutritionand metabolism.com/content/3/1/2>.

94

- A cup of plain hot cocoa (without milk or sugar) has more antioxidants than a cup of tea or a glass of wine.[20]
- Milk chocolate contains several vitamins, including choline, vitamin A, and vitamin K, as well as several minerals, including calcium, magnesium, phosphorus, and potassium.[21]
- Caffeine and theobromine found in chocolate may provide energy, elevate mood, or both.
- Chocolate may be useful in suppressing coughs due to the fact that it contains theobromine.[22]
- Polyphenolic substances in cocoa, and therefore probably in dark chocolate (over 70% cocoa), may decrease LDL (bad) cholesterol, increase HDL (good) cholesterol, and stop the oxidation of LDL (bad) cholesterol.[23,24]
- Cocoa and chocolate may reduce the risk of cardiovascular disease by reducing the risk of forming blood clots, increasing blood flow in the arteries, lowering blood pressure, and having an anti-inflammatory effect.[25]
- Cocoa may have a beneficial effect on cholesterol levels because it consists mainly of stearic acid and oleic acid. Stearic acid is a saturated fat, but unlike most saturated fatty acids, it does not raise blood cholesterol levels. Oleic acid, a monounsaturated fat, does not raise cholesterol and may even reduce it.[26]

---

[20] Lee, K.W., et al., "Cocoa Has More Phenolic Phytochemicals and a Higher Antioxidant Capacity Than Teas and Red Wine," *Journal of Agriculture and Food Chemistry,* 2003; 51(25): 7292-7295.

[21] U.S. Department of Agriculture, ARS, 2008, USDA National Nutrient Database for Standard Reference, Release 21, <http://www.ars.usda.gov/nutrientdata> (December 12, 2008).

[22] http://www.fasebj.org/cgi/content/full/19/2/231 PERMISSIONS

[23] Baba, S., et al., "Plasma LDL and HDL Cholesterol...,"*The Journal of Nutrition,* June 2007, 137: 1436-1441, <http://jn.nutrition.org/ cgi/content/full/137/6/1436> (December 4, 2008).

[24] Wan, Y., et al., "Effects of cocoa powder and dark chocolate on LDL oxidative susceptibility and prostaglandin concentrations in humans," *American Journal of Clinical Nutrition,* November 2001, 74(5): 596-602, <http://www.ajcn.org/cgi/content/abstract/74/5/596> (December 4, 2008).

[25] See footnote 19.

[26] University of Michigan Integrative Medicine, Healing Foods Pyramid, "Dark Chocolate," 2009, <http://www.med.umich.edu/UMIM/food-pyramid/dark_chocolate.htm>.

Cons:

- High fat content.
- Caffeine in chocolate may cause headaches, anxiety, insomnia, heart palpitations, high blood pressure, digestive problems, or urinary tract disorders, and can promote dehydration.[27] It may also aggravate hypoglycemia and fibrocystic breast disease. (Dark chocolate is generally higher in caffeine than milk chocolate. White chocolate is generally caffeine free.)
- Tyramine (a naturally occurring amino acid) in chocolate may cause migraine headaches in sensitive individuals.
- Oxalates in chocolate may promote the formation of kidney stones in those prone to them.[28]
- Caffeine and theobromine, which are both found in chocolate, have been shown to cause severe testicular atrophy (reduced testicle size) in laboratory animals.[29]
- Milk may interfere with the absorption of antioxidants in chocolate.[30]
- Conventionally produced chocolate and chocolate products may contain residues from applied pesticides, herbicides, fungicides, rodenticides, or other chemicals (or a combination of these).
- The theobromine and caffeine in chocolate can be deadly to dogs, cats, and other animals when ingested.

7. Coffee

Pros:

- May help prevent diabetes.[31]

---

[27] See footnote 26.

[28] National Institutes of Health, "Kidney Stones in Adults," *Publication #08-2495*, October 2007, <http://kidney.niddk.nih.gov/kudiseases/pubs/stonesadults/index.htm#oxalate> (December 4, 2008).

[29] Friedman, L., et al. Testicular atrophy and impaired spermatogenesis in rats fed high levels of the methylxanthines caffeine, theobromine, or theophylline. *Journal of Environmental Pathology, Toxicology, and Oncology.* Jan-Feb 1979; 2(3): 687-706.

[30] See footnote 26.

[31] Harvard Medical School, "Coffee Health Benefits: Coffee may protect against disease," *Harvard Health Publications, February 2006,* <http://www.health.harvard.edu/press_ releases/coffee_health_benefits.htm> (December 12, 2008).

- Contains antioxidants, with medium-dark roasted brews appearing to have the highest levels.[32]
- The caffeine in coffee may provide energy, elevate mood, or both, and may enhance physical endurance.[33]
- While the caffeine in coffee can have a mild diuretic effect on the body, it is not likely to cause dehydration, as was previously the long-held belief. The potential for minor fluid loss is offset by the water in the coffee.[34]
- The caffeine in coffee may help to alleviate headaches.
- The caffeine in coffee does not promote persistent high blood pressure, as was previously suspected.[35]
- Coffee may lower blood sugar, protect against cancer (particularly against liver, breast, colon, and rectal cancer), and protect men (but not women) from Parkinson's disease.[36]

Cons:
- Stains teeth and dentures.
- Naturally occurring chemicals (diterpenes called cafestol and kahweol) in coffee beans and some types of brewed coffee prepared without a paper filter (such as lattes and cappuccino) raise cholesterol and triglyceride levels in humans and appear to mildly affect the integrity of liver cells (those at increased risk of heart disease who drink large amounts of coffee should select brews low in diterpenes).[37]

---

[32] Nicoli, M.C., et al., "Antioxidant Properties of Coffee Brews in Relation to the Roasting Degree," *LWT,* May 1997; 30(3): 292-297. Copyright © 1997 Academic Press Limited. All rights reserved.
[33] Committee on Military Nutrition Research, Food and Nutrition Board, Caffeine for the Sustainment of Mental Task Performance: Formulations for Military Operations. Reprinted with permission from the National Academies Press. Copyright © 2001, National Academy of Sciences.
[34] University of Illinois, McKinley Health Center, "Caffeine," October 4, 2006, <http://www.mckinley.uiuc.edu/handouts/caffeine.html> (December 4, 2008).
[35] Myers, M.G., "Effects of caffeine on blood pressure," *Archives of Internal Medicine,* Vol. 148, No. 5, 1189-93, May 1988. Copyright © 1988 American Medical Association. All rights reserved.
[36] See footnote 31.
[37] Urgert, R. and Katan, M.B., "The cholesterol-raising factor from coffee beans," *Journal of the Royal Society of Medicine,* November 1996; 89(11): 618-623.

- Caffeinated coffee can cause anxiety or jitters, insomnia, headaches, nervousness, and other effects.
- The consumption of caffeinated coffee is associated with cardiovascular effects including increased heart rate, increased blood pressure, and occasional irregular heartbeat.[38]
- Researchers have found a link between cholesterol increases and decaffeinated coffee, possibly because of the type of bean being used.[39]
- Caffeinated coffee can be habit forming.
- Decaffeinated coffee can contain caffeine—sometimes in amounts greater than caffeinated coffee.[40] (Caffeine-free coffees generally contain no caffeine.)
- Decaffeinated coffee produced by solvent extraction may contain chemical residues (decaffeinated coffees produced by water extraction are available).
- A reduction in the consumption of caffeinated coffee can cause withdrawal symptoms including headaches, sweating, and nervousness.
- Conventionally produced coffees and coffee products may contain residues from applied pesticides, herbicides, fungicides, rodenticides, or other chemicals (or a combination of these).
- Overconsumption of caffeine due to excessive coffee intake or the cumulative effect of combined caffeine from coffee, other caffeinated beverages, and prescription or over-the-counter drugs, or any combination of these, may cause negative effects on health.[41]
- High caffeine intakes from coffee may increase the risk of toxicity from some drugs, including albuterol (Alupent), clozapine (Clozaril), ephedrine,

[38] Harvard Medical School, "Coffee Health Risks: For the moderate drinker, coffee is safe says Harvard Women's Health Watch," *Harvard Health Publications, August 2004,* <http://www.health.harvard.edu/press_releases/coffee_health_risk.htm> (December 12, 2008).
[39] Harvard Medical School, "Coffee Health Benefits: Coffee may protect against disease," *Harvard Health Publications, February 2006,* <http://www.health.harvard.edu/press_releases/coffee_health_benefits.htm> (December 12, 2008).
[40] Trunk, Denise, "UF experts: decaffeinated coffee is not caffeine-free," *University of Florida News,* October 10, 2006, < http://news.ufl.edu/2006/10/10/decaf/> (December 12, 2008).
[41] Carrillo, J.A. and Benitez, J., "Clinically significant pharmacokinetic interactions between dietary caffeine and medications," *Clinical Pharmacokinetics,* August 2000; 39(2): 127-53.

epinephrine, monoamine oxidase inhibitors (MOIs), phenylpropanolamine, and theophylline.[42]

• Abrupt caffeine withdrawal has been found to increase serum lithium
levels in people taking lithium, potentially increasing the risk of lithium
toxicity.[43]

8. Tea

[**Note:** all varieties of non-herbal tea (white, oolong, green, and black)
come from the leaves of the same evergreen plant, *Camellia sinensis.* Herbal
teas come from a variety of sources.]

Pros:

• Many herbal teas have health benefits when used appropriately.
• Many teas contain antioxidants, known as flavonoids, that may provide
health benefits.
• Epidemiological studies have shown that flavonoid intake is inversely
related to mortality from coronary heart disease and to the incidence of
heart attacks.[44]
• Tea (particularly white tea) may help protect the body from the effects
of carcinogenic (cancer-causing) compounds formed during the cooking
of meats, fish, and other foods.[45]

Cons:

• Stains teeth and dentures.
• Incorrect use of herbal teas can lead to health problems.

---

[42] Higdon, Jane and Drake, V., Linus Pauling Institute, "Tea," January 2008, <http:// lpi.oregonstate.edu/
infocenter/phytochemicals/ tea/index.html#intro> (December 10, 2008).
[43] See footnote 31.
[44] Buhler, D.R. and Miranda, C., "Antioxidant Activities of Flavonoids," November 2000,
<http://lpi.oregonstate.edu/f-w00/flavonoid.html> (December 10, 2008).
[45] Xu, M, et al., "Protection by green tea, black tea, and indole-3-carbinol against 2-amino-3-
methylimidazo[4,5-*f*]-quinoline-induced DNA adducts and colonic aberrant crypts in the F344 rat,"
Carcinogenesis, 1996; 17:1429–1434. Copyright © 1996 Oxford University Press. Reprinted with permission.

- Conventionally produced teas and tea products may contain residues from applied pesticides, herbicides, fungicides, rodenticides, or other chemicals (or a combination of these).
- Teabags made with bleached paper may contain dioxins or other chemicals that can have adverse effects on health.
- Caffeine in tea can cause anxiety or jitters, insomnia, headaches, nervousness, and other effects.
- High caffeine levels in some teas may have adverse health effects.
- Caffeinated tea can be habit forming.
- Decaffeinated tea can contain caffeine (caffeine-free teas generally contain no caffeine).
- Tea contains fluoride, sometimes in high amounts. Excessive tea drinking may cause dental fluorosis (caused by intake of too much fluoride), especially in children.
- Tannin in tea may inhibit nonheme iron absorption in the body.[46]
- Tannin in tea can cause constipation.[47]
- Tea contains **theophylline,** a xanthine stimulant similar to caffeine that may cause insomnia, headaches, or other effects and may cause overdose in those taking prescription theophylline.
- Overconsumption of caffeine due to excessive tea intake or the cumulative effect of combined caffeine from tea, other caffeinated beverages, and prescription or over-the-counter drugs, or any combination of these, may cause negative effects on health.[48]
- High caffeine intake from tea may increase the risk of toxicity of some drugs, including albuterol (Alupent®), clozapine (Clozaril®), ephedrine,

[46] Kim, H., and Miller, D., "Proline-Rich Proteins Moderate the Inhibitory Effect of Tea on Iron Absorption in Rats," *Journal of Nutrition,* March 2005, 135:532-537, <http://jn.nutrition.org/cgi/content/full/135/3/532> (March 11, 2009).
[47] Evidence-based Systematic Review of Green tea (Camellia sinensis) by the Natural Standard Research Collaboration. Natural Standard (www.naturalstandard.com) last accessed 12/10/08. Copyright©2009. Somerville, MA USA.
[48] Harvard Medical School, "Coffee Health Benefits: Coffee may protect against disease," *Harvard Health Publications, February 2006,* <http://www.health.harvard.edu/press_ releases/coffee_health_benefits.htm> (December 12, 2008).

epinephrine, monoamine oxidase inhibitors, phenylpropanolamine, and theophylline.[49]
- Abrupt caffeine withdrawal has been found to increase serum lithium levels in people taking lithium, potentially increasing the risk of lithium toxicity.[50]

9. Wheat

Pros:
- Whole wheat is a very good source of fiber.
- Whole wheat contains naturally occurring vitamins and minerals, including thiamin (vitamin B_1), riboflavin (vitamin B_2), niacin (vitamin B_3), folic acid, vitamin E, calcium, phosphorus, zinc, copper, selenium, and iron. It is also a good source of magnesium and a very good source of manganese.
- Whole wheat provides beneficial fiber for those with diverticulosis, given there are no other contraindications to its use.
- Consuming whole grains reduces the risk of coronary heart disease, may help prevent constipation and hemorrhoids, and may help with weight management.[51]
- Whole wheat provides lutein and zeaxanthin, two carotenoid (vitamin A precursor) nutrients that contribute to eye health and whose consumption is associated with a lower risk of age-related macular degeneration (blindness) and heart disease.[52,53]

---

[49] Urgert, R. and Katan, M.B., "The cholesterol-raising factor from coffee beans," *Journal of the Royal Society of Medicine,* November 1996; 89(11): 618-623.
[50] Carrillo, J.A. and Benitez, J., "Clinically significant pharmacokinetic interactions between dietary caffeine and medications," *Clinical Pharmacokinetics,* August 2000; 39(2): 127-53.
[51] U.S. Department of Agriculture, "Grains," *MyPyramid.gov.,* September 11, 2008, <http://www.mypyramid.gov/pyramid/grains_why_print.html> December 2, 2008.
[52] U.S. Department of Agriculture, ARS, 2008, USDA National Nutrient Database for Standard Reference, Release 21, <http://www.ars.usda.gov/nutrientdata> (December 12, 2008).
[53] Myklebust, M. and Wunder, J., "Eggs," Healing Foods Pyramid, 2009, <http://www.med.umich.edu/UMIM/food-pyramid/eggs.htm> (December 10, 2008).

Cons:
- Common allergen.
- Can harbor disease-causing pathogens including Salmonella, Clostridium perfringens, Clostridium botulinum, Bacillus cereus, and mycotoxins.
- Bleached and bromated wheat has been stripped of most or all of its naturally occurring nutrients.
- Wheat is a gluten-containing grain that causes health problems for those with celiac disease and gluten sensitivity.
- Conventionally produced wheat and wheat products may contain residues from applied pesticides, herbicides, fungicides, rodenticides, or other chemicals (or a combination of these).
- Many products, including bread, muffins, and crackers that state "whole wheat" on the packaging often have small amounts of actual whole grain wheat in them and mainly contain nutrient-stripped counterparts instead.
- Wheat in all forms can be easily infested with insects.

10. Corn

Pros:
- A good source of fiber.
- Low in fat.
- No cholesterol.
- Available in a wide variety of forms, including whole kernel and as chips, cereal, or popcorn.
- Provides several nutrients, including thiamine (vitamin B_1), pantothenic acid (vitamin B_5), manganese, phosphorus, potassium, folate, and vitamin C.
- Contains carotenoids (vitamin A precursors).

Cons:
- Conventionally produced corn and corn products may contain residues from applied pesticides, herbicides, fungicides, rodenticides, or other chemicals (or a combination of these).

- Can harbor pathogens including Escherichia coli, Clostridium botulinum, Clostridium perfringens, Staphylococcus aureus, and Bacillus cereus.
- Popcorn may cause gastrointestinal problems for those who have diverticulosis or active diverticulitis.
- Can contain aflatoxins, a type of toxin known to cause severe toxicity in humans and cancer in laboratory animals.[54]

11. Rice

Pros:
- Brown rice contains many naturally occurring nutrients, including vitamins, minerals, protein, and fiber.
- Good source of carbohydrates.
- Brown rice has an average of 2 to 3 times more fiber than white rice.
- White rice can be beneficial when bland diets are necessary during gastrointestinal illness.
- Rice, including wild rice, is recommended for those with celiac disease due to a lack of gluten.[55]
- Rice milks provide a viable dietary option for those who cannot tolerate dairy milk.

Cons:
- Can be easily infested with insects.
- White rice has less fiber and naturally occurring nutrients than brown rice.
- Conventionally produced rice and rice products may contain residues from applied pesticides, herbicides, fungicides, rodenticides, or other chemicals (or a combination of these).
- Many rice-based packaged products contain high amounts of sodium and chemical additives.

---

[54] Cornell University, Dept. of Animal Science, "Aflatoxins: Occurrence and Health Risks," n.d., <http://www.ansci.cornell.edu/plants/toxicagents/aflatoxin/aflatoxin.html> (December 2008).
[55] National Institutes of Health, "Celiac Disease," *NIH Publication No. 07-4269,* May 2007, <http://celiac.nih.gov/CeliacDiseaseChart.pdf> (December 10, 2008).

12. Oats

Pros:

- A good source of fiber, iron, thiamine (vitamin B$_1$), phosphorus, and magnesium.
- Provide numerous vitamins and minerals.
- Have potential heart health benefits due to soluble fiber that helps remove cholesterol.
- Often tolerated by those with celiac disease.
- Filling and satisfying due to fiber content.
- Provide beneficial fiber for those with diverticulosis, given there are no other contraindications to their use.
- Consuming whole grains reduces the risk of coronary heart disease, may help prevent constipation and hemorrhoids, and may help with weight management.[56]

Cons:

- May not be tolerated by those with celiac disease.[57]
- Can be easily infested with insects.
- Conventionally produced oats and oat products may contain residues from applied pesticides, herbicides, fungicides, rodenticides, or other chemicals (or a combination of these).

13. Soy

Pros:

- A source of carbohydrates, protein, and fat.
- A high-calcium food.
- A complete protein.

---

[56] United States Department of Agriculture, "Grains," *MyPyramid.gov.,* September 11, 2008, <http://www.mypyramid.gov/pyramid/grains_why_print.html> December 2, 2008.

[57] Arentz-Hansen, H., et al., "The Molecular Basis for Oat Intolerance in Patients with Celiac Disease," *PLoS Medicine,* October 2004, 1(1): e1. Published online October 19, 2004.

- Good source of fiber.
- Contains numerous vitamins and minerals.
- High in potassium.
- Is a source of both linoleic and linolenic acid, the two essential fatty acids needed by the human body.
- Fermented soy may significantly improve the ecosystem of the human intestinal tract by increasing the amount of probiotics.[58]
- Derivatives of soy may provide an alternative for postmenopausal women for whom traditional hormone replacement therapy is not an option.[59]
- Soy protein products may offer benefits to women in various life stages. These benefits include improved diet and cardiovascular status; prevention of certain types of cancer; improved health following menopause; obesity prevention and control; and more options for food variety.[60]
- Contains phytic acid, a natural antioxidant found in grains, seeds, and beans (and also the principal store of phosphate in plants), believed to play a role in slowing glucose absorption and possibly having an anticancer effect.[61]
- Genistein (a naturally occurring estrogen in soy) may prove to be useful in the treatment of prostate cancer.[62]
- Soybean oil is cholesterol free.

Cons:
- Common allergen.

---

[58] Cheng, I.C., et al., "Effect of fermented soy milk on the intestinal bacterial ecosystem," *World Journal of Gastroenterology,* February 28, 2005; 11(8): 1225-7,<http://www.ncbi.nlm.nih.gov/ pubmed/15754410> (December 12, 2008).
[59] Petri, Nahas E., et al., "Benefits of soy germ isoflavones in postmenopausal women with contraindication for conventional hormone replacement therapy," *Maturitas,* August 20, 2004; 48(4):372-80. Copyright © 2003 Elsevier Ireland Ltd. Reprinted with permission from Elsevier.
[60] Montgomery, Kristen S., "Soy Protein," *Journal of Perinatal Education,* 2003, 12(3): 42-45, <http://www.pubmedcentral.nih.gov/articlerender.fcgi?artid=1595159> (December 10, 2008).
[61] Natl. Inst. of Environmental Health Sciences, "Soy: Filling in the Gaps," *Environmental Health Perspectives,* n.d., <http://www.niehs.nih.gov/health/docs/soy-gaps.pdf> (December 10, 2008).
[62] Lakshman, M., et al., "Dietary Genistein Inhibits Metastasis of Human Prostate Cancer in Mice," *Cancer Research,* March 15, 2008, Vol. 68: 2024-2032.

- Contains phytic acid and oxalic acid, which can bind to minerals such as calcium and potentially promote deficiencies.
- Soy's potential role in breast cancer risk is uncertain.[63]
- Genistein, the primary naturally occurring estrogen in plants and a major component of soy, has been shown to cause reproductive problems in laboratory mice.[64]
- Genistein may block the body's ability to kill breast cancer cells.[65]
- High intake of soy foods and soy isoflavones may cause lower sperm concentration.[66]
- Conventionally produced soy and soy products may contain residues from applied pesticides, herbicides, fungicides, rodenticides, or other chemicals (or a combination of these).
- Consumption of soy may cause thyroid problems.[67]

14. Eggs

Pros:
- Contain all vitamins except vitamin C.
- Good source of protein, vitamin E, and riboflavin (vitamin B_2).
- Many eggs now contain omega-3 fatty acids (due to flax seed or other natural additives in chicken feed).

---

[63] National Institutes of Health, NCCAM, "Soy," *Publication No. D399,* March 2008, <http://nccam.nih.gov/health/soy/> (December 11, 2008).

[64] National Institutes of Health, NIEHS, "Component in Soy Products Causes Reproductive Problems in Laboratory Mice," *NIH News,* January 10, 2006, <http://www.niehs.nih.gov/news/ releases/2006/ genistein.cfm> (December 12, 2008).

[65] Jiang, X., et al., "Low Concentrations of the Soy Phytoestrogen Genistein Induce Proteinase Inhibitor 9 and Block Killing of Breast Cancer Cells by Immune Cells," *Endocrinology,* 2008; 149(11): 5366-5373, <http://endo.endojournals.org/cgi/content/abstract/en.2008-0857v1> (Dec. 12, 2008).

[66] Chavarro, J.E., et al., "Soy food and isoflavone intake in relation to semen quality parameters among men from an infertility clinic," *Human Reproduction,* 2008; 23(11): 2584-2590. © 2008 by the European Society of Human Reproduction and Embryology. Reprinted with permission from Oxford University Press.

[67] Doerge, D.R. and Sheehan, D.M., "Goitrogenic and Estrogenic Activity of Soy Isoflavones," *Environmental Health Perspectives,* June 2002, Vol. 110, Suppl. 3, <http://www.pubmedcentral.nih.gov/ articlerender.fcgi?artid=1241182> (December 12, 2008).

- Provides numerous minerals, including iron, zinc, calcium, iodine, and selenium.
- Egg yolks provide most of an egg's vitamins and minerals, along with lutein and zeaxanthin, two carotenoid (vitamin A precursor) nutrients that contribute to eye health and whose consumption is associated with a lower risk of age-related macular degeneration (blindness) and heart disease.[68]

Cons:
- Common allergen.
- Can carry Salmonella enteritidis, a foodborne pathogen that may cause gastrointestinal illness especially if the shells are broken, or if eggs or egg products are consumed raw or undercooked.
- Conventionally produced eggs and egg products may contain chemical residues from applied pesticides, processing chemicals, or additives (or a combination of these).[69]
- High in cholesterol, though this may be less of a dietary issue than previously thought.
- A protein in raw egg whites called avidin binds biotin, therefore making biotin unavailable for absorption by the body.

15. Oranges

Pros:
- Contain numerous vitamins and minerals, as well as phytochemicals and flavonoids.
- High in vitamin C.

---

[68] Myklebust, M. and Wunder, J., "Eggs," Healing Foods Pyramid, 2009, <http://www.med.umich.edu/UMIM/food-pyramid/eggs.htm> (December 10, 2008).
[69] Podhorniak, Lynda V., et al., "A Collaborative Effort Between the U.S. Environmental Protection Agency, the Food and Drug Administration, and the University of Arkansas to Develop a Method for the Determination of Part Per Billion Levels of Carbamate Pesticide Residues in Eggs," 2005, *EPA Science Forum*.

- Good source of folate.
- High in fiber.
- Provide antioxidants and enzymes.
- Contain no cholesterol.
- Fat free.

Cons:
- The peels of conventionally produced oranges, which are often used to make candies, jams, marmalades, and other products, may contain residues of fungicides, artificial color (Citrus Red No. 2), or other chemicals or additives including wax or shellac.
- Conventionally produced oranges and orange products may contain residues from applied pesticides, herbicides, fungicides, rodenticides, or other chemicals (or a combination of these).

16. Dairy Products (Milk, Cream, Cheese, Half & Half, Ice Cream, Sour Cream, Yogurt, Butter)

Pros:
- High in protein.
- Good sources of calcium.
- Good sources of lysine, which may aid those with herpes simplex.
- Full-fat, lowfat, and nonfat versions are available.
- Sources of conjugated linoleic acid (CLA).
- Many dairy products, including various types of milk and yogurt, contain lactobacillus acidophilus and lactobacillus bifidus, two digestive aids known to enhance intestinal health.

Cons:
- Many are high in fat.
- Mucous forming.

- Common allergen.
- Can cause unpleasant gastrointestinal symptoms for those who are lactose intolerant.
- Conventionally produced dairy products may contain chemical residues from antibiotics, hormones, processing agents, or the application of pesticides, herbicides, fungicides, or rodenticides (or a combination of these). They may also contain chemical additives.
- Smoked cheeses can contain a variety of carcinogens (cancer-causing agents), especially in the rinds.[70]
- Consumption of low fat milk by males may be a risk factor for prostate cancer.[71]
- Consuming raw milk or cheese made from raw milk may result in serious illness or death.[72]

17. Oils

Pros:
- Many oils provide health benefits.
- Can aid in healthy weight gain.
- Many oils, including flaxseed (linseed), canola, sunflower, soybean, olive, perilla, hemp, safflower, corn, and cottonseed oil, provide essential fatty acids.
- Fatty acids in oils help promote healthy skin.[73]

---

[70] Guillén, M.D. and Sopelana, P., "Occurrence of polycyclic aromatic hydrocarbons in smoked cheese," *Journal of Dairy Science,* March 2004; 87(3): 556-64.

[71] Torniainen, S., et al., "Lactase persistence, dietary intake of milk, and the risk for prostate cancer in Sweden and Finland," *Cancer Epidemiology Biomarkers & Prevention,* May 2007, 16(5): 956-61, <http://www.ncbi.nlm.nih.gov/pubmed/17507622> (December 11, 2008).

[72] U.S. Food and Drug Administration, "FDA and CDC Remind Consumers of the Dangers of Drinking Raw Milk," *FDA News,* March 1, 2007, <http://www.fda.gov/bbs/topics/NEWS/2007/ NEW01576.html> (December 11, 2008).

[73] Boelsma E., Hendriks, H.F., and Roza, L., "Nutritional skin care: health effects of micronutrients and fatty acids," *American Journal of Clinical Nutrition,* 2001; 73(5): 853-864, <http://www.ajcn.org/cgi/content/abstract/73/5/853> (December 11, 2008).

Cons:
- Processing, bleaching, and deodorizing can deplete an oil's nutrients.
- Overuse can lead to unwanted weight gain.
- Many oils have a low smoke point and are not stable under high heat.
- Can go rancid; rancid oils can cause health problems.
- Conventionally produced oils may contain residues from applied pesticides, herbicides, fungicides, rodenticides, or other chemicals (or a combination of these).
- Omega-6 supplements may induce seizures in those who have seizure disorders.[74]
- Some types of oils and oil supplements interact negatively with certain medications.

18. Peanuts & Peanut Butter

Pros:
- Contain carbohydrates, protein, and fat, as well as numerous vitamins and minerals.
- Contain phytosterols (plant-based compounds similar to cholesterol that inhibit intestinal absorption of cholesterol[75]).
- Good sources of protein.
- Contain omega-6 fatty acids.
- Good sources of folate and vitamin E.
- Biopesticide (natural pesticide) use has been shown to successfully reduce the incidence of aflatoxin (a toxic metabolite caused by specific fungi) contamination on peanuts.[76]

---

[74] Evidence-based Systematic Review of Evening primrose oil by the Natural Standard Research Collaboration. Natural Standard (www.naturalstandard.com) last accessed 12/13/08. Copyright©2009. Somerville, MA USA.

[75] Higdon, J. and Drake, V., "Phytosterols," September 2008, <http://lpi.oregonstate.edu/infocenter/phytochemicals/sterols/> (December 11, 2008).

[76] Dorner, J.W., "Control of aflatoxins in peanuts," May 31, 2006, *American Chemical Society Abstracts,* <http://www.ars.usda.gov/research/publications/Publications.htm?seq_no_115= 198380> (December 11, 2008).

Cons:
- Common allergen.
- Can contain aflatoxins, toxic metabolites known to cause severe toxicity in humans and cancer in laboratory animals.[77]
- Conventionally produced peanuts and peanut products may contain residues from applied pesticides, herbicides, fungicides, rodenticides, or other chemicals (or a combination of these).

19. Potatoes

Pros:
- Provide carbohydrates and protein.
- Good source of fiber.
- Provide numerous vitamins and minerals, including thiamin (vitamin B_1), riboflavin (vitamin B_2), niacin (vitamin B_3), pyridoxine (vitamin B_6), calcium, magnesium, zinc, folate, phosphorus, and iron.
- High in vitamin C and potassium (a baked potato with its skin has more potassium than a banana).
- Fat free.
- Cholesterol free.

Cons:
- When cooked at temperatures above 248 °F (120 °C) can contain high levels of acrylamide, a probable human carcinogen (cancer-causing agent).[78] This includes potato chips and French fires.
- Contain solanine, a naturally occurring glycoalkaloid toxin, which can be detrimental to health at high levels such as those found in the leaves and stems of nightshade family plants (e.g., tomato, eggplant, potato, tobacco) and whose presence may be indicated by greening under a potato's skin

---

[77] Cornell University, Dept. of Animal Science, "Aflatoxins: Occurrence and Health Risks," n.d., <http://www.ansci.cornell.edu/plants/toxicagents/aflatoxin/aflatoxin.html> (December 2008).
[78] National Cancer Institute, "Acrylamide in Food and Cancer Risk," July 29, 2008, <http://www.cancer.gov/cancertopics/factsheet/risk/acrylamide-in-food#ques7> (December 11, 2008).

(though potato tubers are tested for their level of glycoalkaloids by the USDA prior to commercial release for sale).[79]

- Some varieties, including already naturally red sweet potatoes, may be processed with artificial red dye to make them appear even redder.[80] Regulations for dyeing potatoes vary by state.
- Conventionally produced potatoes and potato products may contain residues from applied pesticides, herbicides, fungicides, rodenticides, or other chemicals (or a combination of these).

20. Soda

Pros:

- Ginger ale, preferably organic, can be useful during certain types of chemotherapy (shaken down first to lessen bubble content) given that there are no contraindications to its use.

Cons:

- Can contribute to the incidence of dental caries (cavities).
- Generally high in sugar.
- Provides empty calories (generally has little nutritional value).
- Conventionally produced sodas may contain processing chemicals or chemical additives (or a combination of these).
- May have different ingredients depending on whether it is sold at the supermarket or on tap.
- Cola consumption may contribute to lower bone mineral density in older women, a condition that increases the risk of osteoporosis.[81]

---

[79] Pavlista, A., "Greening," *Potato Education Guide,* n.d., <http://www.panhandle.unl.edu/potato/ html/greening.htm> (December 11, 2008).

[80] U.S. Food and Drug Administration, "Sec. 585.825 Sweet Potatoes-Dyeing of Yellow and Red Varieties," November 29, 2005, <http://www.fda.gov/ora/compliance_ref/cpg/cpgfod/ cpg585-825.htm> (December 11, 2008).

[81] Tucker, K.L, et al., "Colas, but not other carbonated beverages, are associated with low bone mineral density in older women: The Framingham Osteoporosis Study," *American Journal of Clinical Nutrition,* Vol. 84, No. 4, 936-942, Oct. 2006, <http://www.ajcn.org/cgi/content/abstract/84/4/936>.

- Caffeinated soda can be habit forming.
- Are often chronically consumed in the diet in place of more nutritious beverages.

21. Cane Sugar

Pros:
- Adds flavor to a variety of foods, beverages, condiments, candies, and gums.
- May act as a preservative at high concentrations.
- Is an alternative to synthetic sweeteners.

Cons:
- Can contribute to dental caries (cavities).
- Generally provides empty calories (little or no nutrients).
- Conventionally produced sugars may contain residues from applied pesticides, herbicides, fungicides, rodenticides, or other chemicals (or a combination of these).
- Consumption must be carefully regulated or avoided by those with diabetes and hypoglycemia.

22. Fried Foods

Pros:
- Frying may lock in nutrients in certain foods.
- Fast preparation.

Cons:
- Generally have a high fat content.
- May be prepared in oils that are not stable under heat.
- Often contain trans fat.
- Can be difficult to digest.

- Can cause indigestion and acid stomach.
- May promote obesity, acne, and other health conditions.
- Many fried foods contain acrylamide, a probable human carcinogen.[82]
- The application of high heat to conventionally produced foods that contain chemical residues from processing, additives, or the application of pesticides, herbicides, fungicides, or rodenticides (or a combination of these) may create additional chemicals, which may in turn have negative effects on health.

23. Pasta

Pros:
- Source of carbohydrates and protein.
- Whole grain types offer fiber in addition to naturally occurring nutrients.
- Fortified pastas provide vitamins and minerals.
- Whole grain pasta provides beneficial fiber for those with diverticulosis, given there are no other contraindications to its use.
- Consuming whole grain pasta reduces the risk of coronary heart disease, may help prevent constipation and hemorrhoids, and may help with weight management.[83]

Cons:
- Can be easily infested with insects.
- Pasta made from refined grain is generally low in fiber.
- Conventionally produced pasta products may contain residues from applied pesticides, herbicides, fungicides, rodenticides, or other chemicals (or a combination of these).

---

[82] National Cancer Institute, "Acrylamide in Food and Cancer Risk," July 29, 2008, <http://www.cancer.gov/cancertopics/factsheet/risk/acrylamide-in-food#ques7> (December 11, 2008).
[83] United States Department of Agriculture, "Grains," *MyPyramid.gov.,* September 11, 2008, <http://www.mypyramid.gov/pyramid/grains_why_print.html> December 2, 2008.

24. Alcoholic Beverages

Pros:
- May reduce risk of coronary artery disease.[84]
- Various studies have shown potential health benefits associated with wine consumption.
- Resveratrol (a natural compound found mainly in the skins of red grapes), antioxidants, and other factors in wine may provide health benefits.
- Beer generally contains small amounts of minerals, some vitamins, and certain amino acids.

Cons:
- High calorie content (7 calories per gram).
- Negatively interacts with many medications.
- Acetaldehyde and many other chemicals that form in the body due to alcohol ingestion have damaging health effects, including the likely potential to cause cancer.[85]
- The consumption of alcohol may promote colorectal cancer.[86]
- Red and white table wines have a high fluoride content.[87]
- Wine may contain high levels of potentially hazardous metal ions such as lead.[88]

---

[84] Klatsky, Arthur L., et al., "Red Wine, White Wine, Liquor, Beer, and Risk for Coronary Artery Disease Hospitalization," *American Journal of Cardiology,* August 15, 1997; 80(4): 416-420. © 1997 Elsevier Science Inc. Reprinted with permission from Elsevier.
[85] U.S. Environmental Protection Agency, "Acetaldehyde," January 2000, <http://www.epa.gov/ttn/atw/hlthef/acetalde.html> (December 11, 2008).
[86] Cho, Eunyoung, et al., "Alcohol Intake and Colorectal Cancer: A Pooled Analysis of 8 Cohort Studies," *Annals of Internal Medicine,* April 20, 2004; 140(8): 603-613, <http://www.annals.org/cgi/content/abstract/140/8/603> (December 12, 2008).
[87] U.S. Department of Agriculture, ARS, 2008, USDA National Nutrient Database for Standard Reference, Release 21, <http://www.ars.usda.gov/nutrientdata> (December 12, 2008).
[88] Naughton, D.P., and Petroczi, A., "Heavy metal ions in wines: meta-analysis target hazard quotients reveal health risks," *Chemistry Central Journal,* October 30, 2008; 2:22, <http://www.journal.chemistrycentral.com/content/2/1/22> (December 11, 2008).

- Conventionally produced alcoholic beverages may contain residues from applied pesticides, herbicides, fungicides, rodenticides, or other chemicals (or a combination of these).
- Alcoholic beverage consumption is listed as a "known human carcinogen" in the National Institutes of Health Report on Carcinogens, 11th Edition. The Report states that consumption of alcoholic beverages is causally related to cancers of the mouth, pharynx, larynx, and esophagus, and goes on to say that studies indicate that the risk is most pronounced among smokers and at the highest levels of consumption. The Report reports that the effect of a given level of alcoholic beverage intake on cancers of the head and neck is influenced by other factors, especially smoking, but that smoking does not explain the increased cancer hazard associated with alcoholic beverage consumption. The Report also states that there is evidence that suggests a link between alcoholic beverage consumption and cancer of the liver and breast.

25. Cereal

Pros:
- Quick and easy to prepare.
- A good source of carbohydrates and protein.
- Fortified cereals provide numerous nutrients.
- Unrefined whole grain cereals provide complex carbohydrates as well as naturally occurring vitamins, minerals, and fiber.
- Many cereals are cholesterol free.
- Consuming whole grains reduces the risk of coronary heart disease, may help prevent constipation, and may help with weight management.[89]

Cons:
- Can be easily infested with insects.

---

[89] United States Department of Agriculture, "Grains," *MyPyramid.gov.*, September 11, 2008, <http://www.mypyramid.gov/pyramid/grains_why_print.html> December 2, 2008.

- Many cereals are made with bleached and bromated grains, as well as degermed grains, all of which are lower in fiber and naturally occurring nutrients than whole grains.
- Many cereals contain artificial colors, flavors, and preservatives and other chemical additives.
- Cereals made with gluten-containing grains (namely wheat, barley, and rye) need to be avoided by those with celiac disease or gluten sensitivity.
- Conventionally produced cereals and cereal products may contain residues from applied pesticides, herbicides, fungicides, rodenticides, or other chemicals (or a combination of these).

Chapter 5

Over 65 million American adults—roughly 29 percent—are currently on a diet.[1] In addition, a large and growing number of the nation's children and adolescents are also on diets. From the young to the middle-aged, the diet craze is in full swing. Yet despite the number of programs, plans, and products available to help us shed pounds, and the amount of money being spent on them—an estimated $55.4 billion in the United States in 2006 alone, with most purchases made by U.S. consumers[2]—the overall incidence of overweight and obesity in this country has continued to grow. During the six-year period from 1999 to 2004 the number of overweight children and adolescents and obese men increased significantly.[3] Between 2003 and 2004 alone an estimated 17.1% of children and adolescents between the age of 2 and 19 (over 12 and a half million) were overweight, and 32.2% of adults (over 66 million) were obese, while nearly 5% of adults were extremely obese.[4]

One factor in the escalation of overweight and obesity is the increasing availability of food. We are consuming more food and more calories than in the past. The USDA's Economic Research Service (ERS) reports that the amount of food available annually for each person in the country rose from 1,675 pounds in 1970 to 1,950 pounds in 2003, while at the same time calorie intake increased from 2,234 calories to 2,757 calories per person daily.[5]

---

[1] Calorie Control Council, "New Survey Reveals Dieting A Constant Concern," August 9, 2007, <http://www.caloriecontrol.org/pr_08092007-b.html> (December 20, 2007).

[2] LaRosa, John, "U.S. Weight Loss and Diet Control Market," Marketdata Enterprises, Inc., <www. marketdataenterprises.com> April 16, 2007. For further info visit www.bestdietforme.com.

[3] Ogden, Cynthia L., Carroll, Margaret D., Curtin, Lester R., McDowell, Margaret A., Tabak, Carolyn J., and Katherine M. Flegal. "Prevalence of Overweight and Obesity in the United States, 1999-2004." *JAMA*, Vol. 295, No. 13. Copyright © 2006 American Medical Association. All rights reserved.

[4] See footnote 3.

[5] Hodan, Farah and Buzby, Jean, United States Dept. of Agriculture, ERS, Amber Waves, "U.S. Food Consumption Up 16 Percent Since 1970," November, 2005, <http://www.ers.usda.gov/AmberWaves/November05/Findings/USFoodConsumption.htm> (March 1, 2006).

Other potential factors include inactivity, genetics, changes in metabolism, specific diseases (e.g., hypothyroidism, Cushing's syndrome, and polycystic ovary syndrome), smoking cessation, insufficient sleep, and the effects of certain medications.[6]

The Typical American Diet

The typical American diet, often referred to as the Standard American Diet (S.A.D.), is high in fat, salt, sugar, and chemical additives and low in fiber. It often leads to obesity and a host of nutrition-related diseases, many of which can be life threatening. Part of the problem is that in our fast-paced society we often opt for the convenience of fast foods, the majority of which fall short of providing optimal nutrition. Many of us consume these foods for breakfast, lunch, and dinner on a daily or near-daily basis, often in the form of oversized portions. We also tend to overeat to avoid wasting food versus wasting food to avoid overeating.

Another part of the problem is our insatiable desire for the taste of foods that have less nutritional value than others. Flavor, in fact, steers many of our decisions about food. The irony here is that many substantially healthy foods are delicious—we simply have never tried them or have tried one we didn't like and then decided to forgo trying any others, regardless of how they are prepared.

Still another part of the problem lies in the fact that for many of us, the amount of energy we expend each day does not match or even come close to the amount of calories we consume. As a result we often shift from consuming the standard American diet to dieting.

---

[6] National Institutes of Health, NIDDK, "Understanding Adult Obesity," *NIH Publication No. 06–3680*, November 2008, <http://www.win.niddk.nih.gov/publications/understanding.htm# causes> (December 12, 2008).

Other Types of Diets

In addition to the standard fare consumed by many Americans there are a number of established diets followed in society. Here are the most common of them:

Vegetarian Diets

Vegetarian diets consist mainly of fruits, vegetables, grains, legumes, nuts, and seeds. They may or may not include eggs, milk, or other dairy products. The American Heart Association also recognizes a *semi-vegetarian diet,* which doesn't include red meat but does include chicken and fish in addition to plant foods, dairy products, and eggs.

The *lacto-ovo vegetarian diet* (lacto is Latin for milk; ovo for eggs) consists mainly of fruits, vegetables, grains, legumes, nuts, and seeds, along with milk and eggs. Variations of this diet include the *lacto vegetarian diet,* in which milk and other dairy products are consumed but eggs aren't, and the *ovo vegetarian diet,* in which eggs are consumed but milk and dairy products aren't. The latter is often opted for among those who are lactose intolerant or have sensitivities to dairy products.

The *vegan* or *total vegetarian diet* is the strictest form of vegetarianism. This type of diet includes only plant-based foods.

Cultural Diets

These diets encompass many unique and traditional foods and dishes, as well as cultural food restrictions, from different regions of the globe including South America, Europe, the Middle East, Asia, and the Mediterranean.

Medical Diets

A wide variety of diets make up this category, including those for cancer, diabetes, colitis, celiac disease, diverticulitis, pregnancy, arthritis, alcoholism, and a host of other diseases and conditions. Some are for weight loss; others are for weight gain. Still others are designed to alleviate symptoms or promote a cure.

Weight Loss Diets

There are over fifty publicly recognized weight loss diets and dozens of others that are less well known, with new ones constantly being introduced. Some are based on calorie intake, others restrict the consumption of fat, carbohydrates, or protein, or any combination of the three. Others involve portion control, regulated eating times, food combining, fasts, or the use or restriction of specific fruits and vegetables. Still others involve the use of foods that are low on the glycemic index (a scale that ranks how quickly specific foods raise our blood sugar level—for additional information see **http://lpi.oregonstate.edu/infocenter/foods/grains/gigl.html**), chemical-free foods, or foods believed to be most beneficial for us based on our blood type. There are also exchange plans, vinegar diets, olive oil diets, diets that require the use of low-energy-density foods (foods that are low in fat and high in nutrients, such as fruits and vegetables), and others.

Some diets incorporate the use of foods that contain indigestible fats, such as Proctor & Gamble's Olestra (also known by its brand name Olean®) or pills that block fat absorption, such as GlaxoSmithKline's allī.™ Each of these has effects that should be considered before their use. Olestra, according to Proctor & Gamble, can absorb the fat-soluble vitamins A, D, E, and K and keep the body from absorbing them. The company adds a small amount of these vitamins to products that contain Olestra to offset this effect. Olestra can also affect the uptake of some carotenoids (vitamin A precursors) from foods because they are fat-soluble, though the company notes that the FDA does not require products made with Olestra to be supplemented with carotenoids since there is currently a lack of scientific agreement on whether they actually provide a health benefit. When eaten in large amounts Olestra may cause abdominal cramping and loose stools, while allī can cause loose stools, more frequent stools that may be hard to control, or gas with an oily discharge if too much fat is consumed during a meal. Those who are on certain medications or who have gastrointestinal problems may encounter other effects or more dramatic effects from these products.

Weight Control Diets

Similar to weight loss diets though often less restrictive, weight control diets are generally part of overall weight control plans that incorporate exercise and other factors for weight maintenance.

Weight Gain Diets

Often utilized by those trying to build muscle or recuperate from illness, these diets focus on higher calorie intake through a well-balanced eating plan that includes a combination of complete proteins, beneficial fats, and unrefined carbohydrates.

Climbing The Pyramids

In addition to the various types of diets, there are numerous resources that provide dietary recommendations as they relate to nutrition and health. Several of these resources offer guidance in the form of "pyramids" that denote suggested, and often conflicting, dietary approaches. Among them is the USDA's MyPyramid Plan, which was designed to help people achieve good eating habits, a healthy weight, and better overall health through diet and physical activity. Although the plan includes updates and additional information over its precursor, the USDA Food Guide Pyramid of 1992, many still find it to be lacking in overall accuracy and ease of use. One such person is Walter C. Willett, M.D., author of *Eat, Drink, and Be Healthy: The Harvard Medical School Guide to Healthy Eating,* who, together with faculty members in the Harvard School of Public Health, designed an alternative pyramid in 2001 developed from numerous years of experience and a wide variety of research avenues. Like the USDA's version, Dr. Willett's "Healthy Eating Pyramid" is not a one-size-fits-all answer to nutrition. It is not intended to be. Rather, it is a regularly updated, research-based set of guidelines for the average healthy person that, according to Willett, is more accurate, complete, and easier to use than the USDA pyramid, is more adaptable to individual needs, and has more of a focus on long-term health.

Other useful evidence-based guides for healthy eating include the Asian,

Latin, Mediterranean, and vegetarian pyramids promoted by Oldways Preservation and Exchange Trust. While Willett's Healthy Eating Pyramid was developed utilizing even more extensive research than each of these, they do offer the benefit of focusing on specific cultural and choice-related issues. However, they too must be adapted to individual needs. Given the fact that we have gender differences, cultural requirements, varied activity levels, and specific genetic patterns, and may be affected by allergies, sensitivities, or medical conditions, there is virtually no way that any food pyramid—or any diet, eating plan, or nutritional program, for that matter—can be an exact fit for everyone.

Good Food & Bad Food

Current modes of thought maintain that there are no good foods or bad foods, only foods. There are good and bad choices, however. For the majority of us, continually eating a diet loaded with fat, salt, sugar, and chemical additives that is also devoid of fruits, vegetables, and whole grains is unlikely to help us maintain an ideal weight and a good level of overall health. By reading labels and learning how to decipher them we also become better able to recognize the nutritional value of specific foods and make healthier choices. Many experts emphasize that total calorie intake should be our main focus when making food selections, and that that intake should come from a variety of healthy food sources.

The Appestat: Our Hunger Meter

Feeling hungry is our body's signal that a void needs to be filled. This signal, which is believed to be regulated by an area of the brain often referred to as the appestat, is our body's call not only for calories, but also for nutrients. A distinct example is when a woman craves laundry starch, ice, or dirt during pregnancy, a condition known as pica. These unusual cravings are a direct indication that the body is making a demand for specific nutrients. Similarly, when we eat an abundance of foods that do not meet our body's nutritional requirements or which create additional nutrient needs (such as refined white flour and sugar), we may crave certain foods or find that we are hungrier than usual, or both. This is both the body's message to us that its nutrient needs are not met and its way of attempting to get us to fill them. Unfortunately when hunger returns we often eat more of the same less-nutritious foods or more of the foods that create additional nutrient needs. This common cycle can lead to overeating and subsequent weight gain, and may be more pronounced if we are not taking appropriate nutritional supplements to fill the nutrient void.

These considerations help us to see that when we are overweight it isn't necessarily a reduction in food intake that is necessary, but rather a change in the types of foods being consumed. Learning about foods and how to prepare them aids us in selecting and creating meals that are not only satisfying to our palates, but also adequate for our body's nutritional requirements.

The Truth About Diet Secrets

While numerous weight loss-related ads and articles would have us believe otherwise, in actuality there are no diet secrets. Rather, there is one simple formula that applies to our bodies for most of our lives: calories taken in combined with an equal amount of calories expended will keep us at relatively the same weight, and in most cases, in better overall health—especially if those calories are derived from nutritionally substantial sources. While there are several variable factors that can affect this equation, including growth, injuries, illness, pregnancy, hormonal imbalances (rarely), and the effects of certain medications, this is generally the case. When people refer to diet secrets they are usually referring to their own tactics (or someone else's) that help them lose weight. In effect these are individualized diet strategies—some of which are sensible and effective and include the consumption of nutritious foods—and others that are unhealthy and should literally be kept a secret.

Stubborn Pounds Are Stubborn For A Reason

When most of us go on a diet there comes a point, usually somewhere between a few weeks and several weeks into dieting, at which weight loss slows down considerably, or stops completely. This is the body's reaction to

125

what it views as an attack or injury. The technical term for this effect is diet-induced adaptive thermogenesis. Because the body uses fat for insulation, hormone regulation, and other essential functions, it attempts to shield itself against excessive fat loss. It is also likely to become more effective at storing fat after we lose it. In addition, while we are losing fat, we are also losing calorie-burning muscle tissue and nutrients. The body attempts to protect itself from these losses as well.

Dieting is commonly associated with recurrent weight gain, often past the initial weight that promoted dieting in the first place. Extreme dieting (following diets that provide less than 800 calories per day) has the potential to result in heart rhythm abnormalities, which can be fatal.[7] Beginning a heavy workout program at the same time may increase this risk. Rapid weight loss (more than 3 pounds per week after the first couple of weeks) may increase our risk of developing gallstones.[8] Rapid or considerable fat breakdown may also have other effects on our bodies. In mammals, including humans, fat is the storage site for chemicals. Just as hormones, antibiotics, and other chemicals harbor themselves in the fat of meat and poultry, chemicals we ingest are stored in our body fat, where they may reside for very long periods.[9] Given these considerations, and when losing weight quickly is not a medical necessity, losing it slowly or moderately is generally a more practical tactic.

Ideal Weight

Body weight varies per person given our age, sex, height, and other considerations. Our "ideal" weight is that at which we feel our best and at which we are not at risk of incurring weight-induced medical problems—either from being overweight *or* underweight. While the topic of what designates ideal weight is somewhat controversial and is often linked to how we look,

---

[7] National Institutes of Health, NIDDK, "Weight loss and Nutrition Myths," August 2006, <http://win.niddk.nih.gov/publications/myths.htm#dietmyths> (December 11, 2008).
[8] See footnote 7.
[9] Centers For Disease Control and Prevention, Agency For Toxic Substances and Disease Registry, "Public Health Statement for Chlordane," Updated October 2007, <http://www.atsdr.cdc.gov/toxprofiles/phs31.html> (December 29, 2007).

the most commonly used criteria for determining a healthy weight is our Body Mass Index, or BMI. BMI is a formula based on height and weight that helps both men and women determine an approximate healthy weight. The National Institutes of Health provides both a BMI calculator and BMI data tables at **http://www.nhlbisupport.com/bmi/**. BMI results are currently categorized as follows:

- Underweight = <18.5
- Normal weight = 18.5-24.9
- Overweight = 25-29.9
- Obesity = BMI of 30 or greater

Eating Right vs. Dieting

Eating right is relative to each of us, our metabolism, our gender, and our state of health. It means eating sufficient but not overwhelming quantities of quality, nutrient-rich, fiber-filled foods that benefit our body's metabolism; help bolster our immune system and protect us against illness; help us maintain a good energy level; and provide us with overall physical and mental well-being. It also means avoiding foods that don't agree with us and lessening or eliminating our intake of foods that have little nutritional value. Once we learn how to make balanced food choices that meet our body's nutritional demands without increasing our weight (unless that's our goal), our chances of improving our health or avoiding health problems increases —sometimes dramatically. At minimum, we often just plain feel better.

Dieting, on the other hand, may or may not incorporate what our individual bodies see as eating right. This depends on the type of diet used, how restrictive it is and in what ways, and other factors. Unlike learning to eat right and incorporating a consistent pattern of healthy eating using a variety of foods without rigorous restrictions, dieting often requires substantial changes that are quite restrictive. As a result many people give up on a diet, later trying the same diet again with the same results, or trying a different diet altogether. And the cycle continues.

A Better Approach

In many cases, extreme dieting and restrictive diets backfire, leaving us frustrated and even more prone to overeating and gaining additional weight. Changing what we eat and losing weight more slowly allows the body more adjustment time, which often results in permanent weight loss—especially when other beneficial lifestyle changes are implemented at the same time. The body sees the slower weight loss as an adjustment rather than an assault.

There are also other things we can do to assist ourselves in losing and maintaining weight, many of which have a behavioral basis. For example, when the temptation to eat an abundance of a food that has little nutritional value hits us or is prompted by irresistible ads or commercials, we can practice the "mind over flavor" technique of making dietary choices. This is done by considering whether we can buy or make a healthier and equally good or better tasting version of the food, and if we can't, by either choosing not to eat it or eating a moderate amount of it, keeping our health in mind. When ads or commercials tempt us to indulge (or overindulge) in such foods we can also consider our health and tell ourselves, "I won't be sold. I can make a better choice. I'm worth it. I win."

A Changing Perspective On Dieting

While the percentage of adult Americans on diets actually *fell* from 33 percent in 2004 to 29 percent in 2007, the number of attempts at dieting increased.[10] This may indicate that some consumers have given up dieting altogether while others have put their weight loss efforts into overdrive. It is more likely, however, that a growing number of us have come to realize the benefits of making consistent lifestyle changes with regard to nutrition and have begun to implement those changes in place of dieting, while others are trying harder than ever to make dieting work for them. Unfortunately many of us try a weight loss plan, program, or product, then give up and try another one in what all too often ends up being an endless and

---

[10] Calorie Control Council, "New Survey Reveals Dieting A Constant Concern," August 9, 2007, <http://www.caloriecontrol.org/pr_08092007-b.html> (December 20, 2007).

128

costly effort to lose weight. We try pills, patches, powders, and plant roots; fat burners, fillers, and fiber, all to little or no avail. Making lifestyle changes that involve diet and exercise generally offers a healthier, more permanent,

and often less costly solution. Consider that when we are seriously over-weight, medical intervention often includes the same common denominators that we employ when we are slightly overweight: to change what we eat and expend more energy through a sensible exercise program. A person who undergoes gastroplasty to decrease the size of their stomach and re-duce their appetite is often given similar, if not identical, diet and exercise recommendations post-surgery.

All in all, concentrating more on what makes up our diet and less on restricting our diet is likely to lead to a better understanding of nutrition, improved eating habits, and enhanced overall health.

Chapter 6

*C*arbohydrates, proteins, and fats are macronutrients (nutrients needed by the body in larger amounts than others) that are essential to life and good health. They each perform specific vital functions in the body and provide us with energy in the form of calories. In this chapter we take a closer look at them, from which foods contain them to which types are best to consume or avoid.

Carbohydates

Carbohydrates are the body's primary energy source, supplying energy to our cells more quickly than either protein or fat. They consist of carbon, hydrogen, and oxygen. They are derived mainly from plant foods and break down in our bodies in the form of glucose, which is essential for brain function. Any available glucose that is not used for our immediate energy needs is stored in our liver and muscles in the form of glycogen, where it is readily retrieved by the body as needed.

Fiber is an exception. While most types of fiber are technically carbohydrates in themselves in addition to being a part of other carbohydrates, their structure is built in such a way that the body can't break them down into glucose. Some types (cellulose and lignin) are completely indigestible—and that's a good thing. Instead of causing a rise in blood sugar, they help to stabilize it. Both the soluble (dissolvable in water) and insoluble (not dissolvable in water) forms of fiber in foods aid our digestive tract and provide us with other health benefits when eaten in moderation.

Types of Carbohydrates
There are two main types of carbohydrates: simple and complex. Simple carbohydrates are among the components that make up complex carbohydrates. They are also found in refined foods, often in abundance, while

complex carbohydrates generally aren't (an example of an exception is when whole oats are added to the top of a loaf of refined bread). Of the two types, complex carbohydrates offer a higher level of nutritional benefits. Here's a basic overview:

Simple Carbohydrates. Simple carbohydrates, also called simple sugars, include monosaccharides (from Greek "mono" and Latin "saccharum," meaning "one sugar") and disaccharides (sugars made from two monosaccharides). They lack the fiber and nutrients found in complex carbohydrates. They also tend to be digested more quickly than complex carbohydrates (though not in all cases), which causes sharp, rapid increases in blood sugar levels.

Dietary **monosaccharides** are:

- *glucose,* also called *dextrose* in the past (found in many foods; especially fruit and honey);

- *fructose,* also called *levulose* (found mainly in fruit and honey, though also in some vegetables); and

- *galactose* (found mainly in milk and dairy products).

Dietary **disaccharides** are:

- *maltose,* found mainly in grains and in lesser amounts in corn syrup (composed of two glucose molecules combined);

- *sucrose,* also known as table sugar, found in sugar cane, sugar beets, fruits, vegetables, and honey (one glucose molecule and one fructose molecule combined); and

- *lactose,* also called milk sugar (one glucose molecule and one galactose molecule combined).

Many refined foods contain large amounts of simple carbohydrates. This includes products made with refined wheat flour (including unbleached flour), processed starchy foods such as white rice and fries, candy, most forms of sugar, and all sugar alcohols (sweeteners chemically derived from sugar). The mechanical and chemical refinement processes these foods undergo generally cause them to lose most or all of their naturally occurring fiber and nutrients. Manufacturers often add one or both of these back in a different form. When this occurs the products are referred to as being enriched or fortified.

Complex Carbohydrates. Complex carbohydrates are found in whole fruits, vegetables, grains, and legumes (beans and peas). They are a combination of:

- *simple and complex sugar molecules* (any combination of monosaccharides, disaccharides, oligosaccharides, and polysaccharides);

- *fiber;* and

- *micronutrients* (essential vitamins, minerals, and other nutrients needed by the body in small amounts).

Some complex carbohydrates, namely grains and certain vegetables, also provide amino acids.

Carbohydrates & Dieting
Many diets restrict carbohydrate consumption. Most involve carbohydrate counting as we commonly know it. Some, however, are based on counting "net carbs" or "impact carbs" (two terms developed and used by the food industry that have not been approved for use by the FDA). These are described as the remaining carbohydrates in foods after fiber, sugar alcohols, and any other types of carbohydrates that are known or believed to have a negligible impact on blood sugar have been deleted. There is controversy over the effectiveness of using this approach for dieting.

133

A moderate reduction in carbohydrate intake combined with the consumption of complex carbohydrates in place of those that are refined can help us feel full and lose weight. Extreme carbohydrate reduction, however, can have a variety of negative effects on health, ranging from headaches and sluggishness to ketosis (the accumulation of chemicals called ketones in the bloodstream that results when the body is required to use fat, rather than carbohydrates, for energy) and bone problems.[1] For diabetics, diets that are both low in carbohydrates and high in protein may increase the risk of kidney damage, exacerbate existing kidney disease, or lead to diabetic ketoacidosis, a life-threatening emergency condition.[2] The USDA's current recommendation for carbohydrate intake for adults and children over the age of four is 45 to 65 percent of our recommended total daily calorie intake[3]— that's between 900 and 1300 calories based on a 2000-calorie diet. They also recommend consuming 14 grams of fiber for every 1000 calories consumed.[4]

Many of the highest carbohydrate foods and beverages have been refined or processed. They include pastries, pies, cakes, cookies, doughnuts, breads, bagels, waffles, breakfast bars, sweetened fruits and vegetables, candy, ice cream, high-sugar alcoholic beverages, most cereals, and all high-sugar non-alcoholic drinks, including sodas and sweetened teas. They also include numerous fast foods.

Carbohydrates contain 4 calories per gram. Alcohol, a simple sugar made from fermented carbohydrates, contains 7 calories per gram. Unlike most other foods it is absorbed in the stomach as well as in the small intestine. Alcohol not only adds a significant amount of calories to the diet, but also releases numerous toxins into our systems that require the liver and other

[1] "Low carb diets may stress body too much, studies find," Arizona State University, December 2007, <http://www.poly.asu.edu/news/2007/12/06/>.
[2] "The Dangers of High-Protein, Low-Carbohydrate Diets for People With Diabetes," Adapted from the 2002 edition of the Johns Hopkins Diabetes White Paper, <http://www.hopkinshospital.org/health_info/Diabetes/Reading/highprotein.html> (December 11, 2008).
[3] U.S. Dept. of Agr., "Carbohydrates," *Dietary Guidelines for Americans 2005*, July 9, 2008, <http://www.health.gov/dietaryguidelines/dga2005/document/html/chapter7.htm> (December 11, 2008).
[4] U.S. Dept. of Agriculture, CNPP, "2005 Dietary Guidelines for Americans," *Backgrounder,* <http://www.cnpp.usda.gov/Publications/DietaryGuidelines/2005/2 005DGBackgrounder.pdf> (December 12, 2008).

organs to work overtime in an effort to filter them out and eliminate them from the body.

Proteins

Proteins play major roles in the structure, function, and regulation of cells within the body. They serve as enzymes, hormones, receptors, and transporters as well as antibodies against disease. Without them we would not be able to breathe, think, or move, let alone grow, digest foods, heal wounds, or reproduce.

Types of Proteins

Proteins are the building blocks of cells; amino acids are the building blocks of proteins. There are over 20 amino acids used by the body, 9 of which are generally considered essential (clinical viewpoints vary on this number), which means we must obtain them from our diet. They are: histidine isoleucine, leucine, lysine, methionine, phenylalanine, threonine, tryptophan, and valine. Among the others are those that are "nonessential" (these are made by the body, mainly in the liver, and our bodies can also manufacture them from other amino acids obtained in our diet) and those that are often referred to as "semi-essential," or "conditionally essential" depending on the stage of life we are in, our state of health, or both. They include: alanine, arginine, asparagine, aspartic acid, cysteine, glutamic acid, glutamine, glycine, proline, serine, and tyrosine.

Proteins that contain all 9 essential amino acids are called "complete" proteins; those that don't are referred to as "incomplete" proteins. Animal sources of protein such as meat, milk, and eggs generally provide all 9 essential amino acids and are complete proteins, while most vegetable sources are lacking a sufficient amount of at least one essential amino acid and are considered incomplete. Two foods that are commonly eaten and are exceptions to this general rule are gelatin and soy. Gelatin is an animal source of protein that lacks two essential amino acids—tryptophan and methionine,[5]

---

[5] "Gelatin," McGraw-Hill Concise Encyclopedia of Science and Technology, Fifth Edition, © 2005.

making it an incomplete protein. Soy, on the other hand, is a vegetable protein that provides *all* of the essential amino acids, making it a complete protein.[6] We can create complete proteins by combining foods, such as eating beans with rice or vegetables with pasta.

Protein & Dieting

Diets that are high in protein are often low in carbohydrates, and vice-versa. While they are frequently touted as a good way to lose weight fast, their long-term safety and effectiveness have yet to be proven. Extreme restriction of carbohydrates or excessive intake of protein may have the potential to lead to negative health effects, especially in those who are in moderately poor to substantially poor health, though more research needs to be done in this area.

On a more positive note, protein requires more calories to burn than either carbohydrates or fat. This is due to the fact that it takes the body more effort to break it down. However, adequate consumption, rather than excessive consumption, is likely to be the best bet.

Like carbohydrates, protein provides 4 calories per gram. The recommended daily intake for adults and children over 4 years of age is 50 grams per 2,000 calories of food eaten.[7] This equates to just over 7 grams of protein per 20 pounds of body weight on a daily basis.[8] The Reference Daily Intake (RDI) for protein for infants under 1 year is 14 g; for children 1 to 4 years, 16 g; for pregnant women, 60 g; and for nursing mothers, 65 g.

For more information on protein visit:
http://www.cdc.gov/nutrition/everyone/basics/protein.html

---

[6] Henkel, John, "Soy: Health Claims for Soy Protein, Questions About Other Components," *FDA Consumer Magazine,* May-June 2000, <http://www.fda.gov/Fdac/features/2000/300_ soy.html> (December 11, 2008).

[7] Kurtzweil, Paula, "'Daily Values' Encourage Healthy Diet," n.d., < http://www.fda.gov/FDAC/special/foodlabel/dvs.html> (December 12, 2008).

[8] USDA Center for Nutrition Policy and Promotion, "2005 Dietary Guidelines for Americans," *Backgrounder,* <http://www.cnpp.usda.gov/Publications/DietaryGuidelines/2005/2005DG Backgrounder.pdf> (December 12, 2008).

Fats

Fats, also referred to as lipids, are made up of fatty acids. They contain 9 calories per gram, more than twice the amount provided by either carbohydrates or protein. For the most part, they are seen as a negative factor that should be avoided in our diets. But in reality many of them are assets to our health. The key is to eat beneficial fats, and to eat them in moderation.

Fats in general have several essential functions in our bodies. For example, they transport the fat-soluble vitamins A, D, E, and K through the bloodstream and, together with bile acids from the liver, aid in their absorption in the small intestine.[9] They also provide essential fatty acids that our bodies need but can't make on their own, help regulate bodily processes, protect our vital organs, and insulate our nerves. And fats provide an especially important source of calories for people who are underweight and for infants and toddlers up to 2 years of age, who have the highest energy needs per unit of body weight of any age group.[10]

Types of Fat

There are three main types of dietary fat: unsaturated, saturated, and trans. They are each made up of carbon, hydrogen, and oxygen, though their names are derived solely from how the carbon and hydrogen atoms found in each type are configured (see Figure 1). They come from both plant and animal sources and exist in various combinations in foods in the form of triglycerides (three fatty acids hooked to a glycerine molecule). Some are chemically altered. Here's a basic overview of them:

---

[9] Bowen, R., "Secretion of Bile and the Role of Bile Acids in Digestion," *Pathophysiology of the Digestive System, The Liver: Introduction and Index,* November 2001, <http://arbl.cvmbscolostate.edu/hbooks/pathphys/digestion/liver/bile.html> (April 5, 2007).

[10] U.S. Food and Drug Administration, "Olestra and Other Fat Substitutes," *FDA Backgrounder,* November 1995, <http://vm.cfsan.fda.gov/~dms/bgolestr.html> (December 12, 2008).

Unsaturated Fats: The "Good" Fats

Unsaturated fats, also called unsaturated fatty acids, are those that contain at least one carbon atom that is double bonded (has two attachments) to another carbon atom. Each double bond has two less hydrogens than a single bond (see Figure 1), making the fatty acid it appears in "unsaturated" with hydrogen (saturated fats have only single carbon bonds). When these unsaturated fats are in their natural "cis" formation and have not been chemically altered into trans fats (also see Figure 1) they help to lower our low-density lipoprotein (LDL) or "bad" cholesterol levels and raise our high-density lipoprotein (HDL) or "good" cholesterol levels when we consume foods that contain them. They also do not promote the development of plaque on the walls of our arteries. There are two types of unsaturated fats:

Monounsaturated Fatty Acids (MUFAs). These fatty acids contain *only one* carbon-to-carbon double bond. Also called ***omega-9 fatty acids***, they are derived from plant foods. Good dietary sources of these fatty acids include olive, canola, soybean, and peanut oils, most nuts and seeds, and avocados.[11]

Polyunsaturated Fatty Acids (PUFAs). These fatty acids contain *more than one* carbon-to-carbon double bond. There are two main groups: ***omega-3 fatty acids*** and ***omega-6 fatty acids***. Each of these groups contain a number of different fatty acids including one **essential fatty acid** that the body can't manufacture on its own and which we must therefore obtain from our diet. These are **alpha-linolenic acid (ALA)** from the omega-3 group and **linoleic acid (LA)** from the omega-6 group. Other nutritionally important omega-3 fatty acids are **eicosapentaenoic acid (EPA)** and **docosahexaenoic acid (DHA)**, while other nutritionally important omega-6 fatty acids are **gamma linolenic acid (GLA)** and **arachidonic acid (AA)**.

Alpha-linolenic acid, along with other omega-3 fatty acids, is found in many plant-based foods including leafy green vegetables, soybeans, walnuts,

---

[11] Harvard School of Public Health, "Omega-3 Fats: An Essential Contribution," *The Nutrition Source,* n.d., <http://www.hsph.harvard.edu/nutritionsource/fats.html>. (December 12, 2008).

flaxseed (an excellent source; also called linseed), and olive oil. It is also found in some types of fish, including salmon, mackerel, and sardines, along with various types of fish oil, though research suggests that obtaining it from fish, rather than fish oil (which is refined), is more beneficial.[12] Linoleic acid, along with other omega-6 fatty acids, is also found in plant-based foods, such as corn, soybean, and safflower oils and evening prim-rose oil. Non-essential omega-6 fatty acids are also present in lesser amounts in animal-based foods including meat, poultry, eggs, and dairy products.

There are seven critical functions of essential fatty acids:[13]

- Developing and maintaining gray matter in the brain
- Achieving optimal growth
- Maintaining the integrity of cell membranes
- Keeping skin healthy
- Supporting proper visual development
- Maintaining a healthy nervous system
- Regulating blood pressure, blood clotting, and the body's inflammatory processes

Saturated Fats: The "Bad" Fats
Unlike unsaturated fatty acids, saturated fatty acids (SFAs) have no carbon-to-carbon double bonds, but rather only carbon-to-carbon single bonds that are fully "saturated" with hydrogen atoms (see Figure 1). They are found in numerous plant- and animal-based foods including meats, most dairy products, egg yolks, cocoa butter, coconuts, coconut oil, palm oil, and palm kernel oil as well as in fish and seafood (especially most fast food and fried

---

[12] Elvevoll, E.O., et al., "Enhanced incorporation of n-3 fatty acids from fish compared with fish oils," *Lipids,* December 2006; 41(12):1109-14.
[13] Boothby, Barbara E., "The Essential Fats of Life," HUHS Nutrition Services, 2004, <http:// huhs.harvard.edu/Resources/HealthInformationByTopic/Nutrition/TheEssentialFatsOfLife.aspx> (March 20, 2007).

versions). These fats have a reputation for raising our harmful LDL cholesterol levels in the blood and contributing to atherosclerosis, heart disease, and other health problems, though there is some controversy over whether the saturated fat found in plant foods (particularly coconut and palm oils) is actually metabolized by the body in exactly the same way as saturated animal fat and has the same overall effects. More research is needed in this area. The American Heart Association currently recommends that saturated fat intake from all sources be limited to less than 7 percent of total daily calories. That's less than 140 calories (approximately 15 grams) of saturated fat per day based on a 2000-calorie diet.

Trans Fats: The Other "Bad" Fats
Trans fats are found mainly in foods that contain partially hydrogenated vegetable oils or have been cooked in them, which includes many stick margarines, commercially prepared baked goods, fried fast foods, candies, and pie crust mixes, and even some "nutrition" bars. They are produced when liquid (unsaturated) vegetable oils are heated and a specific amount of hydrogen is added to them during a process called hydrogenation. Ironically, *fully* hydrogenated oils contain little or no trans fats, though on their own they are too solid for practical dietary use and need to be combined with other oils. Also, although many commercial peanut butters contain partially hydrogenated oils, the small amount added contributes only a miniscule, if even detectable, amount of trans fat to them.[14]

Partially hydrogenated oils were developed to help products maintain their freshness and flavor. The trans fats that result during their production, however, have a negative effect on our bodies by raising the amount of harmful LDL cholesterol in our blood. This type of cholesterol *raises* our risk of developing coronary heart disease. Due to these considerations the American Heart Association recommends that we limit trans fat intake to less than 1 percent of total daily calories (that's just over 2 grams of trans

---

[14] McBride, Judy, "No Trans Fats in Peanut Butter—Contrary to Current Rumor," *ARS News & Information,* June 12, 2001, <http://www.ars.usda.gov/is/pr/2001/010612.htm> (December 13, 2008).

Saturated Fat
(saturated fatty acid)

Unsaturated Fat
(unsaturated fatty acid)
(*cis* fatty acid)

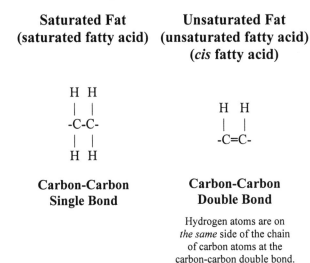

Carbon-Carbon
Single Bond

Carbon-Carbon
Double Bond

Hydrogen atoms are on
the same side of the chain
of carbon atoms at the
carbon-carbon double bond.

Trans Fat
(*trans* fatty acid)

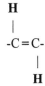

Carbon-Carbon
Double Bond

Hydrogen atoms are on *opposite* sides of the chain of
carbon atoms at the carbon-carbon double bond.

Figure 1. Differences in carbon and hydrogen configuration in dietary fats. *Reprinted with permission from the U.S. Food and Drug Administration.*

fat per day based on a 2000-calorie diet). As of January 1, 2006, the FDA required food manufacturers to list trans fat on the nutrition labels of their products, making it easier for us to do so. However, products with 0.5 g or less of trans fat per serving can be exempted from this requirement, so it is important to be aware that eating multiple servings of foods that contain smaller amounts of trans fat can still cause our trans fat consumption to add up. When in doubt about the actual trans fat content in a product, the FDA recommends contacting the manufacturer.

The Other Side Of The Trans Fat Story

In addition to being found in foods with partially hydrogenated oils, trans fats are also found in animals products, including meat, cream, and butter, though generally in smaller quantities. These particular trans fats, which form in the digestive tract of cows and other grazing animals through inter-actions between bacteria and the omega-6 fatty acid linoleic acid, are re-ferred to as conjugated linoleic acid (CLA).[15] CLA is currently being studied for its potential use in treating cancer and obesity.[16,17]

Cholesterol

While considered a fatty substance rather than an actual fat, cholesterol is another member of the lipid family, from a group of lipids called sterols. It is manufactured in the body, primarily in the liver, though all parts of the body except the brain can make it.[18] It can also be obtained in our diets, though only through the consumption of animal-based foods. Only about 25 percent of the cholesterol in our bodies comes from our diet. While we functionally use cholesterol in the production of bile acids, sex hormones, and cell membranes, having a high blood cholesterol level (a condition

---

[15] "Conjugated linoleic acid (CLA) and weight loss?" *Go Ask Alice!, Columbia University's Health Q&A Internet Resource,* June 3, 2005, <http://www.goaskalice.columbia.edu/3773.html>.

[16] Gaullier, J.M., et al., "Conjugated linoleic acid supplementation for 1 y reduces body fat mass in healthy overweight humans," *American Journal of Clinical Nutrition,* June 2004; 79(6):1118-25.

[17] Smedman, A. and Vessby, B., "Conjugated linoleic acid supplementation in humans—metabolic effects," *Lipids,* August 2001; 36(8):773-781.

[18] Haas, Elson M., <u>Staying Healthy with Nutrition</u>, p. 72, © 2006 Celestial Arts Publishing, Berkeley, CA.

called hypercholesterolemia) can cause an unhealthy buildup of plaque on the walls of our arteries. This is a major risk factor in the development of coronary heart disease (the precursor to heart attacks) and strokes. The presence of large amounts of oxidized cholesterol in the bloodstream is of particular concern. This type of cholesterol is found in fried foods and many other consumables, including dried egg products, powdered milk, cheeses, and a variety of high temperature dried animal products.[19] It can also develop in our bodies due to normal bodily processes.[20] Cholesterol intake should be limited to less than 300 mg per day for most people, however, for those who have coronary heart disease or an LDL cholesterol level of 100 mg/dL or greater, cholesterol intake should be limited to less than 200 milligrams a day.[21]

Fats & Dieting

We often associate eating fat with being fat. This idea holds validity when we consider that fat is more calorie dense than both protein and carbohydrates and eating too much of it can cause us to exceed our caloric requirements. There is also the fact that calories obtained from carbohydrates and protein, respectively, are more readily retrieved by the body for energy needs than those obtained from fat, promoting fat to stay around longer.

Reports on the health risks of excess fat consumption have led to the development of numerous low-fat, reduced fat, and fat-free products. When these products have as many or more calories than their full-fat counterparts, however, they do not effectively help us to lose or maintain weight, especially if we eat them in abundance. The bottom line is that if our calorie intake—be it from fats, protein, or carbohydrates—exceeds our usage and the amount our bodies need to effectively function, the rest is

[19] Hubbard, R.W., Ono, Y., and Sanchez, A., "Atherogenic effect of oxidized products of cholesterol," *Progress in Food & Nutrition Science*, 1989; 13(1):17-44. Copyright © Elsevier 2009.
[20] Engler, Marguerite M., "EARLY Trial: Cholesterol Facts," July 23, 2003, <http://nurseweb.ucsf.edu/public/early./ldl.shtml> (January 18, 2008).
[21] Source: American Heart Association, "Know Your Fats." © 2009 www.americanheart.org.

stored as fat. Thirty-five hundred calories equal one pound, no matter how we obtain them.

Diets that are low in overall fat yet still provide adequate amounts of beneficial fats, complex carbohydrates, and complete proteins represent the optimal way we should eat for life. Eating this way lowers our risk of developing cancer, diabetes, and other common life-threatening diseases. Diets that severely restrict fats or don't provide sufficient amounts of beneficial and essential fats can't provide us with the best level of health. The American Heart Association guidelines urge adults who are trying to lose weight and keep it off to eat no more than 35 percent of total daily calories from overall fat, including less than 7 percent of total daily calories from saturated fat and less than 1 percent of total daily calories from trans fat. That's a maximum of 700 calories derived from fat or approximately 78 grams of fat per day based on a 2000-calorie diet.

Fat Replacers

There are a number of different fat substitutes used in food products in an effort to reduce their overall fat and calorie content. Some are carbohydrate-based, while others are protein-or fat-based. Those that are fat-based include Olestra (brand name Olean®), a nonfat cooking oil used in prepared foods. It is made from ingredients found in common foods such as vegetable oil and sugar. It is neither absorbed nor metabolized by the body, but rather passes through the digestive tract unchanged. All fat-based fat replacers are chemically altered fatty acids or contain them.

Chapter 7

*S*ugars, also called saccharides, come in many forms. Some occur naturally, such as those in fruit and milk, while others, including white table sugar and molasses, are produced commercially from sugar cane and other sources. They are found in a wide variety of both natural and refined foods and beverages. The simplest of these sugars (monosaccharides and disaccharides) exist mainly in fruits, honey, sugar cane, and refined grains and are sweeter than the more complex sugars found in complex carbohydrates. Our taste for the sweetness of sugar in general is innate.

Much of the sugar consumed in the average American diet comes from commercially produced foods and beverages that have had one or more types of sugar added during or after their production to enhance flavor. These "added sugars" are often found in foods and beverages we would not suspect contain them, such as fruit juice drinks, breads, soups, and meat products. The USDA recommends that we consume no more than a total of 40 grams of added sugars (about 10 teaspoons) daily based on a 2000-calorie diet.[1] To assist in this endeavor they provide a useful online database that lists the added sugars content of many common foods. To view it visit **www.ars.usda.gov/Services/docs.htm?docid=12107**. The USDA also provides a comprehensive listing of the total sugar content in many foods at: **www.nal.usda.gov/fnic/foodcomp/Data/Other/herr48.pdf**.

In addition to naturally occurring and commercially produced sugars there are a number of natural and artificial sugar substitutes. Many are used as no-calorie or low-calorie replacements for table sugar and other higher-calorie sweeteners during weight-loss and weight-maintenance programs, while others are used to help avoid the blood sugar fluctuations common to

---

[1] U.S. Department of Agriculture, "Profiling Food Consumption in America, *Agriculture Fact Book,* Chapter 2, n.d., <http://www.usda.gov/factbook/chapter2.htm> (December 12, 2008).

diabetes and hypoglycemia. Manufacturers often use artificial sweeteners in combination with each other (and sometimes with sugars as well) to create high-impact flavor in their products. This is common among both regular and sugar-free gums, some of which contain five different types of artificial sweeteners. Such sweeteners may also be combined to mask bitterness.

As a whole, sweeteners are generally considered to be either nutritive (also called caloric) or non-nutritive (also called non-caloric, alternative, or artificial). Nutritive sweeteners contain calories—4 per gram—while non-nutritive sweeteners are essentially calorie-free.

Our use of sugar and other caloric sweeteners in this country has increased considerably over the past several decades. Between 1970 and 2003 alone the annual per capita consumption of such sweeteners (including cane and beet sugars, edible syrups, honey, high fructose corn syrup, glucose, and dextrose) increased an estimated nineteen percent, from 119 pounds per person in 1970 to 142 pounds per person in 2004.[2] Among these sweeteners, high fructose corn syrup (which is now commonly used in soft drinks) has come under the most scrutiny. Research has shown that its main ingredient, fructose, which is also found naturally in fruit juice, may trigger a hormonal response in our bodies that increases our appetites and promotes weight gain.[3]

Our use of sugar substitutes has also increased. They are found in a wide variety of foods, beverages, and other products including condiments, supplements, and pharmaceuticals. Consumer demand for them in the U.S. is estimated to reach $1.1 billion by 2010.[4]

---

[2] Hodan, Farah and Buzby, Jean, U.S. Dept. of Agriculture, ERS, Amber Waves, "U.S. Food Consumption Up 16 Percent Since 1970," November, 2005, <http://www.ers.usda.gov/AmberWaves/November05/Findings/USFoodConsumption.htm> (March 1, 2006).
[3] Teff, Karen L., et al., " Dietary Fructose Reduces Circulating Insulin and Leptin, Attenuates Postprandial Suppression of Ghrelin, and Increases Triglycerides in Women," *The Journal of Clinical Endocrinology & Metabolism,* 89(6): 2963-2972, <http://jcem.endojournals.org/cgi/content/abstract/89/6/2963> (December 12, 2008).
[4] "U.S. Alternative Sweeteners Demand to Reach $1.1 Billion in 2010," Alternative Sweeteners study from The Freedonia Group, <http://www.freedoniagroup.com>.

The question of which types of sweeteners are best to use depends on a few different factors, including their nutritional value, our state of health, and what they are being used for. In general, the less refined and more natural a sweetener is, the better. Among cane sugar sweeteners, those that are unbleached, unrefined, and organic (or produced in a similar or better manner) are the best choice. Throughout the remainder of this chapter we take a closer look at many of the different types of sugars and sugar substitutes, both nutritive and non-nutritive.

Sugars (Nutritive Sweeteners)

Barley malt
Sprouted or germinated dried barley frequently used to make beer and distilled spirits. Its powdered form is often used in baking. See also *barley malt syrup*.

Barley malt syrup
An extra light to dark syrup derived from sprouted barley grain. It is used in the production of breads, cereals, and other baked goods as well as in the production of beer. Also called malt extract, malt extract syrup, extract of malted barley, malt syrup, dark malt syrup, and malted cereal syrup, it is high in maltose (a disaccharide). It also contains amino acids, protein, vitamins, and minerals including calcium, potassium, phosphorus, and magnesium.[5] Barley malt is also available in powdered form.

Brown rice syrup
Also called rice syrup, rice bran syrup, and rice malt, this versatile gluten-free sweetener is high in both disaccharides (maltose) and polysaccharides (complex carbohydrates). It is used in a variety of foods and products including throat lozenges, candies, cereals, nutrition bars, protein powders,

[5] U.S. Department of Agriculture, ARS, 2008, USDA National Nutrient Database for Standard Reference, Release 21, <http://www.ars.usda.gov/nutrientdata> (December 12, 2008).

and canned goods. It is produced through a process that uses enzymes to break down the starches in brown rice.

Brown sugar

Like white table sugar, brown sugar is produced both from sugar cane and sugar beets. It has more nutrients than white sugar, though like white sugar the amounts it contains are extremely small. Its color is obtained from molasses, though caramel color may also be added. When made from sugar cane it is allowed to maintain a percentage of its naturally occurring molasses; when made from sugar beets, molasses are manually added. **Light brown sugar** contains less molasses than **dark brown sugar** and has a milder flavor. Both are commonly used in baking.

Corn syrup

Derived by processing corn starch with enzymes or acids, this sweetener contains mostly glucose along with some maltose. There are two basic types: light and dark. These descriptions are based only on color. **Light corn syrup** is clear, while **dark corn syrup** has a brown hue that it gets from a combination of refiners' syrup (a type of molasses) and caramel coloring. Both are commonly used in baking and candy making. Other types of corn syrup include **high fructose corn syrup (HFCS)**, in which the glucose derived from the processing of corn starch is further treated to produce fructose, and **high maltose corn syrup (HMCS)**, which is *less* processed than standard corn syrup so as to have a lower glucose level and a higher maltose level. High fructose corn syrup is used in many foods and beverages including breads, candies, soft drinks, jellies, and ketchup. Different preparations of it contain 42%, 55%, or 90% fructose.[6] High maltose corn syrup, also referred to as **maltodextrin**, is used in breads and other baked goods as well as in the production of ice cream and beer. Dark corn

---

[6] Center for Science in the Public Interest, "Food Additives," 2009, <http://www.cspinet.org/reports/chemcuisine.htm> (December 12, 2008).

syrup contains more nutrients than any of the other types, though the amount of nutrients in all of them is extremely small.

Corn syrup solids
A crystallized form of liquid corn syrup. Also called dried glucose syrup, glucose syrup solids, and glucose solids.

Date sugar
A natural dark-colored sweetener consisting of finely ground dried dates. It contains many nutrients (it is a good source of potassium), amino acids, and fiber. Due to the fact that it is an actual fruit that contains fiber, date sugar does not melt the way traditional processed sugars do. Nevertheless, it is used to make many baked goods, including breads, and is added to a variety of foods as a topping or mix-in. It is more expensive than most other sugars.

Dextrose
The scientifically derived name for the most common form of glucose (the dextrorotatory form, which is sweet). The name is no longer in common use and has been replaced simply by "glucose." See also *glucose*.

Fructose
Also called *levulose* or *fruit sugar*, fructose is a monosaccharide derived mainly from fruit and honey, though it is also found in some vegetables. It is the sweetest of the simple sugars, including sucrose (table sugar).

Crystalline fructose, which is used in many foods and beverages, is not made from fruit, but rather is produced by separating the fructose from sugar or cornstarch with the help of enzymes and then allowing the resulting syrup to crystallize.

Galactose
A monosaccharide found mainly in milk and dairy products, though also in some plant-based foods. Some people cannot metabolize this sugar; there

are three disorders associated with its metabolism that are currently being studied.[7]

Glucose

Also referred to as *blood sugar* and previously called *dextrose,* glucose is a monosaccharide sugar found in many foods, especially fruit and honey. It is often produced from corn (also called *maize*) and other starchy plant foods. It is the most commonly consumed form of carbohydrates. See also *glucose syrup.*

Glucose syrup

Also often referred to as corn syrup, glucose syrup is produced by the enzymatic hydrolysis (the breaking of bonds in molecules through the use of enzymes) of starch in corn; though it can also be produced from wheat, potatoes, or other starchy foods. It is also available in dried form. See also *glucose.*

Honey

Honey is a natural sweetener produced mainly by honey bees. Though its composition can vary depending on the floral variety it is derived from, its average nutrient breakdown is 17.1 percent water, 82.4 percent total carbohydrate, 0.3 percent protein, and 0.2 percent fiber.[8] It also contains vitamins, minerals, amino acids, and antioxidants. Its average carbohydrate content is fructose (40.9 percent), glucose (35.6 percent), galactose (3.1 percent), maltose (1.44 percent), and sucrose (0.89 percent).[9]

Honey is available raw or pasteurized, and in liquid or crystallized form. On average it is 1 to 1½ times sweeter than sucrose.[10] It is used in a variety

---

[7] Holton, J.B., "Galactose disorders: an overview," *Journal of Inherited Metabolic Disease,* 1990; 13(4): 476-86. © 1990 Springer Netherlands. With kind permission of Springer Science and Business Media.
[8] U.S. Department of Agriculture, ARS, 2008, USDA National Nutrient Database for Standard Reference, Release 21, <http://www.ars.usda.gov/nutrientdata> (December 12, 2008).
[9] See reference #8.
[10] National Honey Board, "Carbohydrates and the Sweetness of Honey," n.d., <http://www.honey.com/downloads/carb.pdf> (December 12, 2008).

of foods and beverages including baked goods, candies, egg nogs, teas, and salad dressings.

Because honey can contain Clostridium botulinum (botulism) spores, no form of it should be given to infants or children under one year of age.

Invert sugar

Invert sugar is produced by splitting sucrose molecules into their component monosaccharides, glucose and fructose, with the help of an enzyme or acid. This process is referred to as inversion. Invert sugar is sweeter than sucrose and is often used in syrups and candies. Honey is a natural invert sugar made with the help of enzymes provided by bees.

Lactose

Also called milk sugar, lactose is a disaccharide composed of one glucose molecule and one galactose molecule combined and is much less sweet than sucrose. Like galactose, it is one of the only sugars derived from an animal source. It is broken down by lactase, an enzyme that we begin to produce less of after about age 2.[11] Many people are what is termed "lactose intolerant," in which the ingestion of milk (and in many cases dairy products in general) causes them to experience indigestion, gas, bloating, nausea, or diarrhea, or any combination of these symptoms. Lactose intolerance should not be confused with a milk allergy, which can cause itching, sneezing, hives, wheezing, and other typical allergy symptoms and has the potential to be life threatening.

Liquid sugar

Any of a variety of mainly commercial sugar syrups made by either hydrolyzing sucrose or inverting glucose with enzymes.

---

[11] National Institutes of Health, "Lactose Intolerance," *NIH Publication No. 06-2751,* March 2006, <http://digestive.niddk.nih.gov/ddiseases/pubs/lactoseintolerance/> (December 12, 2008).

Malt extract/malt syrup

Although malt combinations made from barley and corn are often referred to as malt extract or malt syrup, the FDA designates that the word "malt" be used solely for products that contain only barley.[12] See *barley malt syrup.*

Malt sugar

See *maltose.*

Maltodextrin

A starch-based, gluten-free powdered sweetener generally made from corn, rice, or potato starch, though it can also be derived from wheat, barley, rye, or other starchy grains.[13]

Maltose

Also called malt sugar, maltose is a disaccharide made up of two glucose molecules. It is found mainly in sprouted grains (including barley, which is used to process beer and distilled spirits) and in smaller amounts in standard corn syrup.

Maltose syrup

Any starch-based syrup derived from grain that contains moderate to high amounts of the disaccharide maltose.

Maple syrup

Made from the sap of sugar maple trees (and also red maple trees),[14] maple syrup is available in different grades, colors, and flavors. It is commonly used as a pancake and waffle topping as well as in candies, salad dressings, and

---

[12] U.S. Food and Drug Administration, Code of Federal Regulations, Title 21, Vol. 3, April 1, 2008, <http://www.accessdata.fda.gov/scripts/cdrh/cfdocs/cfcfr/CFRSearch.cfm?fr=184.1445>.

[13] U.S. Food and Drug Administration, "Gluten-Free Foods: Consumption Patterns and Purchasing Practices of Consumers with Celiac Disease," Slide 21, August 19, 2005, <http://www.cfsan.fda.gov/~dms/glutlee/glulee21.htm> (December 12, 2008).

[14] Blumenstock, B. and Hopkins, K., "How to Tap Maple Trees and Make Maple Syrup," *Bulletin #7036,* n.d.,<http://www.umext.maine.edu/onlinepubs/PDFpubs/7036.pdf>.

other foods, and is also available in granulated and powdered forms. It is high in sucrose and low in glucose. It contains ten minerals and is a good source of calcium and potassium.[15] The USDA grades maple syrups as follows:[16]
Grade A includes light, medium, and dark amber. It must have good color, flavor, and odor, be practically free from defects, and be practically clear. It is commonly sold to consumers. Grade B is for reprocessing rather than retail sales, and must have fairly good color, flavor, and odor, be fairly free from defects, and be fairly clear. Syrups that do not meet the qualifications for reprocessing are considered substandard and are not to be sold to consumers.

Molasses

There are a number of different types of molasses, including those derived from citrus, beets, and wood. The most common forms used by consumers, however, are those obtained from the processing of sugar cane. They include fancy, unsulphured, sulphured, and blackstrap molasses. *Fancy molasses* is produced specifically from crushed sugar cane, while *sulphured*, *unsulphured*, and *blackstrap* molasses are made from residual cane juice obtained during the production of table sugar. *Sulphured molasses* is made from young sugar cane treated with sulphur as a preservative, bleaching agent, or both. *Unsulphured molasses* is made from mature sugar cane and is processed without the use of sulphur. *Blackstrap molasses*, which may be either sulphured or unsulphured, is obtained from the third of three boilings of residual sugar cane syrup and is darker and more robust in flavor than the molasses produced from the first two boilings. The first boiling produces the sweetest molasses.

While sweetness can vary, molasses is generally highest in sucrose, with near equivalent amounts of glucose and fructose.[17] It also contains many nutrients, including calcium, magnesium, and potassium.

---

[15] U.S. Department of Agriculture, ARS, 2008, USDA National Nutrient Database for Standard Reference, Release 21, <http://www.ars.usda.gov/nutrientdata> (December 12, 2008).

[16] U.S. Department of Agriculture, "USDA Quality Standards," February 11, 2008, <http://www.ams.usda.gov/standards/mplesirp.pdf> (December 12, 2008).

[17] U.S. Department of Agriculture, ARS, 2008, USDA National Nutrient Database for Standard Reference, Release 21, <http://www.ars.usda.gov/nutrientdata> (December 12, 2008).

Powdered sugar

Finely ground or crushed granulated sugar used mainly in baked goods, icing, and candy. It often contains a small percentage of corn starch. Two types commonly used by consumers are 10X and 4X; 10X being more finely ground and 4X being coarser. Also called *confectioner's sugar.*

Raw sugar

Sugar that has not been refined. In the U.S., some sugars that have been minimally refined or minimally processed are referred to as raw sugars. One example is Sucanat® (which stands for SUgar CAne NATural), a minimally refined evaporated sugar made from pure cane juice. Another minimally refined sugar is demarara sugar. Also see *turbinado sugar.*

Refinery syrup

A byproduct of refined syrup.[18] Used as part of other syrups and sweeteners as well as in baked goods, candy, sauces, and other foods. Also called *refined sugar syrup* and *refiner's syrup.*

Sorghum syrup

A sweetener extracted from sorghum grass that is often used in place of cane sugar. It is a source of calcium, magnesium, potassium, and other nutrients.[19]

Sucrose

Also known as table sugar, sucrose is found in sugar cane, sugar beets, fruits, vegetables, and honey. It consists of one glucose molecule and one fructose molecule combined. In the form of granulated sugar it contains extremely small amounts of calcium, iron, potassium, selenium, fluoride, and riboflavin (vitamin B-2).[20]

---

[18] U.S. Department of Labor, "Employment in Ginning of Cotton and Processing of Sugar Beets, Sugar-Beet Molasses, Sugarcane, or Maple Sap into Sugar or Syrup," CFR title 29, Chapter V, Part 780, Subpart I, n.d., <http://www.dol.gov/dol/allcfr/ESA/Title_29/Part_780/ 29CFR780.816.htm> (December 12, 2008).
[19] U.S. Department of Agriculture, ARS, 2008, USDA National Nutrient Database for Standard Reference, Release 21, <http://www.ars.usda.gov/nutrientdata> (December 12, 2008).
[20] See footnote 19.

Turbinado sugar
Steamed, unrefined raw sugar that is tan to light brown in color and has larger crystals than table sugar. Also called turbinated sugar.

Wort syrup
Syrup high in glucose or maltose that is generally used in breweries.

Sugar Substitutes

Polyols (Sugar alcohols)
Polyols, also called sugar alcohols, are chemical derivatives of sugar. They include sorbitol, xylitol, mannitol, maltitol, lactitol, and erythritol as well as isomalt and hydrogenated starch hydrosylates. They contain less calories than sugar and do not promote tooth decay. Foods and products they are found in include gum, candy, ice cream, baked goods, throat lozenges, and breath mints. When consumed in large quantities, polyols can cause gastrointestinal distress in the form of cramping, bloating, gas, and diarrhea.

Aspartame (NutraSweet®)
Developed by the NutraSweet Company, aspartame (also commonly known as NutraSweet® and Equal®) is roughly 200 times sweeter than sugar. Although it is often referred to as a no-calorie sweetener, it actually contains 4 calories per gram just like sugar (the FDA allows products with less than 5 calories to be labeled and referred to as "no calorie"). However, it does not cause a rise in blood sugar the way sugar does, nor does it promote tooth decay.

Chemically, aspartame is the methyl ester of aspartic acid and phenylalanine, two amino acids. Methyl esters are organic compounds that turn into methanol in the body. While some foods (including various fruits) and alcohol also contain methanol at what are believed to be safe levels for consumption, there is concern over the amount of methanol ingested among extremely heavy drinkers of aspartame-containing beverages.

Although research has purportedly shown aspartame to be safe for consumption by the general public (except for those with phenylketonuria, also known as PKU, a rare inherited disorder in which the body cannot metabolize phenylalanine and mental retardation and epilepsy can result from its consumption), many people have reported health problems to the FDA after consuming it. The FDA is currently in the process of reviewing data from the European Food Safety Authority (EFSA) regarding a long-term carcinogenicity study of aspartame conducted by the European Ramazzini Foundation which suggests that aspartame is a cancer-causing agent.[21]

Saccharin

Known under the brand names Sweet'N Low,® Sugar Twin,® and Necta Sweet,® saccharin is approximately 300-700 times sweeter than sugar. It is produced synthetically from methyl anthranilate and other chemicals.[22] It contains no calories, does not promote tooth decay, and is heat stable. Although previously listed as a potential cancer-causing agent, the National Toxicology Program determined it should no longer be listed as such in 2000, and as a result Federal legislation allowed the cancer warning to be removed from saccharin labels in 2001. It is used in a wide variety of foods, beverages, and other products, including baked goods, chewing gum, candy, condiments, and animal feed.

Sucralose (Splenda®)

Sucralose is the only sweetener made from cane sugar. It is produced through a patented multi-step process that replaces three hydrogen-oxygen (hydroxyl) groups on a sugar molecule with three chlorine atoms. It is about 600 times sweeter than table sugar and has no calories. Sucralose is not absorbed by the body, but rather passes through the body virtually unchanged.[23]

---

[21] U.S. Food and Drug Administration, "FDA Statement on European Aspartame Study," May 8, 2006, <http://www.fda.gov/bbs/topics/NEWS/2006/NEW01369.html> (December 12, 2008).
[22] U.S. International Trade Commission, "Saccharin From China," *Publication No. 3535,* p.6, September 2002, <http://hotdocs.usitc.gov/docs/pubs/701_731/pub3535.pdf> (March 10, 2009).
[23] Calorie Control Council, "Sucralose Facts," *All About Sucralose,* n.d., <http://www.sucralose.org/brochure05.html> (December 12, 2008).

It was initially approved by the FDA in 1998 for use in 15 food-related categories, and approved for use as a general purpose sweetener in all foods in 1999.

Acesulfame K (Acesulfame Potassium)

Acesulfame K (the K stands for potassium, its elemental letter on the periodic table in chemistry), also called Ace-K and marketed as Sweet One® and Sunett®, is an artificial sweetener that is approximately 200 times sweeter than sugar. It is derived from the processing of acetoacetic acid with potassium.[24] Initially approved by the FDA in 1988 for use in beverages and as a tabletop sweetener, it was approved for general use in foods (except meat and poultry) in December 2003. It is stable under both heat and cold, and is used in baked goods, frozen desserts, candy, beverages, and protein powders. It contains no calories and is not metabolized by the body. Although the Joint Expert Committee on Food Additives (JECFA), which is the scientific advisory group to both the Agriculture Organization of the United Nations and the World Health Organization, has deemed acesulfame K safe for consumption in the amount of 15 mg/kg of body weight per day after reviewing available research, the Center for Science in the Public Interest (CSPI) and others still have concerns over its safety.

Neotame

Produced by the NutraSweet Company, the maker of aspartame, neotame is a high intensity non-nutritive sweetener that is approximately 7,000 to 13,000 times sweeter than table sugar.[25] Chemically similar to aspartame, it was approved by the FDA as a general-purpose sweetener for use in a variety of dietary products in 2002. To date it is not widely used.

---

[24] International Food Information Council Foundation, *Everything You Need to Know About Acesulfame Potassium*, July 1998, < http://www.ific.org/publications/brochures/acekbroch.cfm>.
[25] U.S. Food and Drug Administration, "FDA Approves New Non-Nutritive Sugar Substitute Neotame," *FDA Talk Paper,* July 5, 2002, <http://www.fda.gov/bbs/topics/ANSWERS/2002/ ANS01156.html>.

157

Stevia

Stevia, also called stevioside, is a sweet herb derived from a tropical South American plant. Though it is used in some other countries to sweeten foods and beverages, its safety as a whole has not been proven and the FDA has therefore not approved it for use as a food additive in this country.[26] It is, however, able to be sold as a dietary supplement under provisions of 1994 legislation, so long as it is not promoted as a sweetener. In addition, on December 17, 2008, the FDA granted GRAS (Generally Recognized As Safe) status for high-purity rebaudioside A (rebiana), an ingredient derived from Stevia leaves and marketed as Truvia™ rebiana, for use as a general purpose sweetener, though the status pertains only to high-purity rebaudioside A (rebiana) products that meet the established criteria and not to all stevia.[27]

Tagatose

Approved by the FDA for use as a food additive in October 2003, this naturally occurring sweetener that is chemically similar to fructose is found in dairy products and some other foods, though not in large quantities. It is also commercially produced from whey under the brand name Naturlose.™[28] According to Spherix, which holds patents for uses of Naturlose, it is nearly as sweet as table sugar, has no aftertaste, browns and bakes effectively, doesn't cause blood sugar spikes or tooth decay, and is a prebiotic (inhibits dangerous bacteria and promotes healthy bacteria in the gut). However, since it is poorly absorbed by the body, consuming large amounts of it can cause nausea, flatulence, and diarrhea.[29]

---

[26] U.S. Food and Drug Administration, "Automatic Detention of Stevia Leaves, Extract of Stevia Leaves, and Food Containing Stevia," *Import Alert IA4506*, April 24, 2008, <http://www.fda.gov/ora/fiars/ora_import_ia4506.html> (December 12, 2008).
[27] "Cargill Receives Official Notification From FDA Supporting the Safety of Truvia™ Rebiana," Press Release, December 17, 2008, <www.truvia.com>.
[28] Spherix, " Naturlose Quick Facts," n.d., <http://www.naturlose.com/naturlose-what.htm> (December 12, 2008).,
[29] Center for Science in the Public Interest, "Food Additives," 2009, <http://www.cspinet.org/reports/chemcuisine.htm>.

Chapter 8

*T*he science behind how individual nutrients help us to ward off disease and maintain good health is relatively young. It began to actively evolve just over a century ago after an English doctor by the name of William Fletcher experimented with the diets of residents in an insane asylum and discovered that consumption of unpolished rice (rice with its husk, bran, and germ intact) prevented the disease known as beriberi, while consumption of polished (refined) rice did not. Soon scientists set out to isolate specific active nutritional elements in unpolished rice as well as a variety of other foods, and by the mid 1900s many of the vitamins we use today were discovered. Along the way Polish biochemist Casimir Funk also provided us with the term "vitamine," derived from "vital amine," meaning an ammonia-like substance that was essential for life. The "e" was later dropped from vitamine when it was discovered that not all nutrients were amines, leaving us with the term "vitamin" as we know it today.

Fletcher's work was not the first of its type. Prior to his discovery a number of other important findings were made that linked specific foods with relief from disease, though they failed to set the ball in motion as far as research to uncover individual nutrients was concerned. These include the results of a dietary experiment performed by renowned naval surgeon James Lind in 1747 which proved that an unknown nutrient in citrus fruit (now known as vitamin C) cured scurvy among sailors. They also include similar observations by seaman and explorer Sir Richard Hawkins over a century and a half earlier. Unlike Fletcher's discovery, the findings of both Hawkins and Lind were virtually ignored. It would be nearly another half century after Lind's experiment before citrus would become a provision on ships (earning sailors the name "limeys") and nearly another two centuries before vitamin C would be isolated and named. Today, with advances in research and technology, nutritional science provides us with the ability to more readily investigate and learn about individual nutrients. As a result there are a wider variety of nutritional supplements at our disposal.

Types of Supplements

There are many types of nutritional supplements, most of which are available in different forms (tablets, capsules, chewables, softgels, gelcaps, liquids, sprays, powders, foods, beverages, and, in some instances, injections or intravenous therapy). They include:

- vitamins
- minerals
- enzymes
- phytonutrients (plant extracts)
- amino acids
- antioxidants
- essential fatty acids
- herbs
- glyconutrients (cell communication nutrients)
- probiotics
- prebiotics
- proteins

While these and other nutritional supplements may provide health benefits, they are not food substitutes. In most cases, even those made from whole foods don't provide us with complete nutrition in the form of carbohydrates, fats, protein, fiber, and other dietary essentials.

Are Supplements Really Worth Taking?

"Don't vitamins go right through us?" is a common question asked by consumers. For the most part, the answer is no. Many vitamins (namely the B vitamins and vitamin C) that go "through" our systems are actually used by the body to the extent needed and only any excess is eliminated. This is given that the supplements are of good quality and contain the types and amounts of nutrients listed on the labels. In some cases, however, whole tablets or capsules are eliminated by the body undigested. The potential causes for this include gastrointestinal illness, a lack of sufficient hydrochloric acid, or the effects of inert ingredients such as binders.

One reason for the misconception about the absorbability of supplements in general is that many people think of the intestines as the beginning of waste disposal from the body and nothing more, when they are actually the major sites for nutrient absorption. While alcohol and traditional aspirin (among other things) are actually assimilated in the stomach to some extent, most other foods, drugs, and nutrients are not. The small intestine does most of the assimilation work in each case. Even the colon (part of the large intestine) captures nutrients as the body continues its elimination process.

Another important consideration is the fact that nutrients—be they from healthful foods or beneficial supplements—are likely to help us maintain or improve the health of *all* of our internal organs, including those involved in elimination (our liver, kidneys, bladder, intestines, and colon). Further, while the cost of scientifically proven, high-quality supplements may seem prohibitive, they may in fact help us to ward off diseases such as colon cancer that are far more costly both in terms of money and lives.

Who Needs Additional Nutrients?

If we consume a well-balanced, nutritious diet, obtain adequate sleep, exercise sensibly, keep our stress to a minimum, and avoid toxic chemical exposure (from cigarette smoke, car exhaust, pesticides, and other contaminants), we probably don't need to take additional nutrients. If, however, we don't do these things and our bodies need to work overtime trying to rid themselves of chemicals, heal injuries, protect or repair our immune systems, or deal with underlying health problems, taking additional nutrients is likely to be beneficial. Appropriate nutritional supplementation is likely to benefit those of us who:

- do not eat a well-balanced diet
- are on a vegetarian diet that does not provide all required nutrients (including protein, calcium, zinc, iron, and vitamin B12)
- have serious allergies, sensitivities, or aversions to foods that contain essential nutrients
- are under a great deal of stress
- drink heavily
- smoke
- are ill
- are unable to consume a well-balanced diet
- are highly physically active
- are pregnant
- are injured
- are on a mainly irradiated diet
- have medical conditions that have been proven to benefit from supplemental nutrition

Even when we do consume a well-balanced diet, the foods we choose may provide us with fewer nutrients than we expect due to how they were grown, processed, shipped, packaged, and prepared. For example, food plants often vary in nutritional value simply due to the type of soil they are grown in. Uncultivated natural soil generally contains healthy ratios of minerals and other essentials for plant growth, while cultivated soil is frequently subject to chemicals and overuse, both of which can deplete its available nutrients. The less nutrients there are in soil, the less there are in the foods grown in it.

The mineral content of the water used to grow plant-based foods can also affect their nutritional quality, as can heat, light, cutting, exposure to air, irradiation, and the amount of time that elapses from harvesting to consumption. Boiling or heavily steaming plant-based foods also depletes a percentage of their nutrients (especially those nutrients that are water soluble, such as the B vitamins and vitamin C), and microwaving is likely to have the same effect. Even baking soda and hard water can destroy nutrients in plant-based foods.[1]

How Much Of Each Nutrient Do We Need?

The Dietary Reference Intakes (DRIs) and Adequate Intakes (AIs) of vitamins and minerals vary according to age and gender. They are often highest among women who are pregnant or breastfeeding. The amounts, including their Tolerable Upper Intake Levels (ULs), are set by the Food and Nutrition Board of the National Academy of Sciences. To view them visit **www. iom.edu/Object.File/Master/21/372/0.pdf.**

Why Do Supplements Often Contain Less Or More Than 100% Of The Recommended Daily Value?

The reasons vary and include size restrictions (some types of nutrients take up a good deal of space and may cause a tablet, for example, to be too large to consume), specialized formulas (e.g., for men, women, children), and even marketing ploys to get consumers to buy "sister" supplements in order to get their complete daily nutrients. The percentage of each nutrient included is at the discretion of the manufacturer, therefore contacting a company di-rectly about specific supplements may be useful.

Natural vs. Synthetic

One common question people ask when selecting vitamins is "Should I choose natural or synthetic?" The main consideration behind this question is generally one of bioavailability and quality; in other words, to find out

---

[1] Bastin, Sandra, University of Kentucky, "Vegetable Preparation for the Family," n.d., <http://www.ca.uky.edu/agc/ pubs/fcs3/fcs3106/fcs3106.pdf> (December 13, 2008).

which type will be best absorbed and provide the body with the most benefit. While vitamins that are natural are often derived from foods or plants and may in fact provide us with small amounts of enzymes, phyto-nutrients, or other as-yet undetected beneficial health aspects that their synthetic counterparts do not provide, scientists maintain that for the most part synthetic vitamins are assimilated by the body in much the same way as those that are derived naturally. Two exceptions are natural vitamin E (as d-alpha tocopherol) and folic acid (a synthetically produced form of folate), both of which have been shown to be better assimilated in the body than their synthetic and naturally occurring counterparts, respectively.

Another consideration is the fact that natural food-grade vitamins are generally easy to digest and offer the distinct advantage of being able to be taken on an empty stomach. These two benefits can be useful when nausea presents digestive difficulties (such as during pregnancy when morning sickness is a problem or in other instances of gastrointestinal distress), provided there are no allergies, medication interactions, or other contraindications to their use. Nutrient combinations should be carefully reviewed by a doctor, pharmacist, or other qualified professional before use during pregnancy or when medications are being taken, as some combinations cause serious reactions (also see chapter 14, *Food & Drug Interactions*). Herbs that are sold as supplements or are a component of other supplements may also interact with medications or cause reactions. All herbs should be carefully reviewed before use and avoided where contraindicated.

An additional consideration is that while food-grade supplements are made from food, certain nutrients may still be best absorbed by the body by consuming foods in their natural form. In addition to other factors, the freshness, preparation method, enzyme availability, and overall nutrient content of whole natural foods, both individually and collectively, have the potential to positively affect the bioavailability of food nutrients.

Lastly, it is important to remember that although a supplement may be labeled "natural," not all natural substances are safe or healthy for human (or animal) consumption.

What About Added Nutrients In Foods & Beverages?

Supplemental nutrients that are added to foods, beverages, and meal replacements or are used as preservatives (such as when vitamin E is used to preserve sliced or dried fruit) have the potential to cause an excess or deficiency of one or more nutrients in the body. These situations are dependent upon how much of each particular fortified food is consumed on a regular basis, what type of nutrient is involved, and whether or not additional supplements of the same nutrient are also being consumed.

Since the body's extensive mechanisms do not function based on the effects of only one vitamin, but rather from a synergy combined of many, taking an excess of one nutrient may throw off the ratio of other nutrients in our systems. On the other hand, just because a food, beverage, or other product has added nutrients does not mean those nutrients will be absorbed by the body, especially when one or more nutrient-depleting factors exists in the product itself (e.g., chemical additives or sugar). In some cases added nutrients may not provide any real overall benefit. Also, different forms of nutrients can be either more or less readily absorbed by the body, and our bodies have their own distinct ratios of absorption.

Is It Okay To Take Only One Or Two Supplemental Nutrients On A Regular Basis?

It depends. Just as consuming too much of a food that contains supplemental nutrients has the potential to throw off the body's synergistic nutrient balance, so can taking individual nutrient supplements—especially if other nutrients are lacking in the body at the same time. Generally speaking, taking nutrients individually can pose a number of problems. However, in cases where blood test results show a lack of a specific nutrient or nutrients, and in cases where medication interactions, medical conditions, or surgical considerations are a concern, individual supplementation may be required.

Should Cancer Patients Take Supplements?

The American Cancer Society recommends that cancer patients avoid nutritional supplements. This is due in part to the fact that some supplements, namely antioxidants, may interfere with cancer treatment.[2] For a complete overview on nutritional supplements and cancer visit: **http://www.cancer.org/docroot/ETO/content/ETO_5_3x_How_to_Know_What_Is_Safe_Choosing_and_Using_Dietary_Supplements.asp**.

Can Supplements Be Taken Prior To Surgeries or Medical Procedures?

The consumption of certain supplements in the hours, days, and weeks prior to surgeries and other medical procedures can have serious or even life-threatening effects. Among these supplements are vitamin E and St. John's Wort. All questions regarding the use of supplements should be clearly discussed with the attending physician or surgeon well in advance of surgeries or other procedures.

Who Regulates Nutritional Supplements?

The U.S. Food and Drug Administration (FDA). For detailed information about the FDA's regulatory efforts involving supplements visit **http://www.foodsafety.gov/~dms/supplmnt.html.** For specific information about the marketing of supplements visit **http://www.cfsan.fda.gov/~dms/ds-oview.html#regulate**.

What Are Inert Ingredients In Supplements And How Do They Affect The Body?

[2] D'Andrea, Gabriella M., "Use of Antioxidants During Chemotherapy and Radiotherapy Should Be Avoided," *CANCER,* Vol. 55, No. 5, 2005, pp. 319-321. ©2005 American Cancer Society. This material is reproduced with permission of Wiley-Liss, Inc., a subsidiary of John Wiley & Sons, Inc.

Inert ingredients are those other than the active ingredients in a product. They may or may not have an effect on the body. For example, a synthetic food coloring added to a vitamin tablet is considered an inert ingredient. While one person may experience no noticeable effect from consuming the food coloring, another person who has an allergy to it may experience an allergic reaction.

Inert ingredients may also interact negatively with medications. Further, they may have an effect on the active ingredients within the product itself. In addition to artificial colors, inert ingredients include flavorings, sugar, salt, preservatives, binders, and microencapsulating agents (often used to preserve fish oil), among other substances.

Which Types Of Nutrients Are Best?

Those that...

    ...are fresh (have not passed their expiration date)
    ...are not known to cause adverse effects
    ...do not contain unnecessary or dangerous additives
    ...have not been exposed to extreme temperatures
      (unless required)
    ...have not been exposed to light (if light sensitive)
    ...do not contain heavy metals or pollutants
    ...do not interfere with medications
    ...have proven potencies (by certified laboratory testing)
    ...are backed by sound science and factual marketing
    ...are the correct dosages for our age, gender, and health
    ...are in a form that is easy to digest

See the National Institutes of Health Database at
http://dietarysupplements.nlm.nih.gov/dietary/
to find information on ingredients in over 2000 brands
of dietary supplements.

Is It Beneficial To Buy Supplements In Bulk?

Although cost savings are an incentive, buying supplements in bulk may not be beneficial due to the potential for nutrient or potency loss (or both) that can occur during long-term storage. There is also the possibility that newer, more advanced versions may become available in the interim. Whether buying in person, by phone, or on the internet, confirm expiration dates and ask about any upcoming product changes.

A Look At The Nutrients

The remainder of this chapter provides a **basic overview** of many nutrients that are available to consumers as nutritional supplements, including their various functions in the body, deficiency risks, toxicity information, and food sources.

Vitamins

Vitamins are micronutrients, meaning they are needed by the body only in small amounts. The majority of them must be obtained from plant- or animal-based food sources or from supplements, as they are not manufactured in the body. They fall into two basic categories: water soluble and fat soluble. Water-soluble vitamins (the B vitamins and vitamin C) do not accumulate in the body; when we eat an excess of them we simply excrete them. However, taking high supplemental doses of some of these vitamins—especially niacin and vitamin B_6—can have serious adverse effects. Fat-soluble vitamins (A, D, E, and K), on the other hand, *can* accumulate in the body and cause toxicity and therefore should not be consumed in large or excessive amounts. Here's a basic look at the individual vitamins in these two categories:

Water-Soluble Vitamins

Thiamin (Thiamine, Vitamin B₁)

Thiamin, also called thiamine and vitamin B_1, has many important roles in the body. Like several of the other B vitamins it functions as a coenzyme (an enzyme that assists other enzymes in carrying out their work). It is necessary for brain, heart, muscle, and nerve function. It benefits our nervous and digestive systems, promotes good mental health, and plays an essential part in converting carbohydrates to energy within our cells. It is necessary for the prevention and treatment of beriberi as well as congestive heart failure due to thiamin deficiency.[3] Alcoholics, the elderly, those who are undernourished, and those with chronic illnesses are particularly susceptible to a deficiency of this nutrient, which in severe cases can result in serious complications involving not only the heart, but also the brain (and entire nervous system), lungs, muscles, and gastrointestinal tract.[4] As a deficiency of thiamin can occur in as little as 14 days,[5] those who are on fasting programs or highly restrictive diets for extended periods of time without supplementation are also at risk. Although thiamin is considered to be relatively non-toxic, rare cases of hypersensitivity and serious allergic reactions have been reported, and consumption of high doses may cause dermatitis (skin irritation), drowsiness, or other effects.[6]

Thiamin is destroyed by exposure to heat and air, and can also be lost in the cooking water of boiled and steamed foods, as can all water-soluble vitamins. It is also depleted by a number of enzymes, chemicals, and conditions collectively known as antithiamin factors (ATFs). Among the most common ATFs are enzymes found in many species of raw freshwater and

---

[3] Seligmann, Hanna, et al., "Thiamine deficiency in patients with congestive heart failure receiving long-term furosemide therapy: A pilot study," *American Journal of Medicine,* August 1991, 91(2): 151-155. © 1991 by Excerpta Medica Inc. Reprinted with permission from Elsevier.

[4] Evidence-based Systematic Review of Thiamine by the Natural Standard Research Collaboration. Natural Standard (www.naturalstandard.com) last accessed 12/13/08. Copyright © 2009. Somerville, MA USA.

[5] See footnote 4.

[6] See footnote 4.

saltwater fish and certain species of raw crab and clam, including those that may be used for various types of sushi (this is not a concern with cooked fish and seafood, as these particular enzymes are inactivated by cooking).[7] Tea, coffee, betel nuts, blueberries, and red cabbage also contain ATFs, though the types of ATFs found in these foods are *not* inactivated by cooking.[8]

Dietary Sources Include: Whole grains, wheat germ, sunflower seeds, legumes (beans, peas), nuts, pork, and thiamin-fortified foods and beverages.

Riboflavin (Vitamin B₂)

Riboflavin, also known as vitamin B_2, plays vital metabolic roles in the body and is required for proper cell function and the production of energy. It is also necessary for growth and the development of red blood cells. Riboflavin is used in the treatment of jaundice in newborns, and may be useful in the treatment of many other conditions and disorders, though further research is needed.[9] Riboflavin deficiency, called ariboflavinosis, may present itself in the form of cracked skin or sores at the corners of the mouth; dermatitis (skin rash or irritation); a swollen throat or tongue; anemia; or weakness, among other things.[10] Individuals who are susceptible to a deficiency of this vitamin include alcoholics, the elderly, and those with chronic illnesses. Riboflavin is destroyed by exposure to light and can leach into water during the boiling or steaming of foods.

Riboflavin obtained from both food and supplements is considered to be non-toxic. Excess supplemental riboflavin in the body is simply excreted

---

[7] Berdanier, Carolyn D., CRC Desk Reference for Nutrition, Second Edition, p. 451, Copyright © 2005 CRC Press, Boca Raton, Florida.
[8] Grosvenor, Mary B. and Smolin, Lori A. Nutrition From Science To Life. p. 294. ©2002 Harcourt, Inc. Reproduced with permission of John Wiley and Sons, Inc.
[9] Evidence-based Systematic Review of Riboflavin by the Natural Standard Research Collaboration. Natural Standard (www.naturalstandard.com) last accessed 12/13/08. Copyright © 2009. Somerville, MA USA.
[10] See footnote 9.

in the urine, usually causing the urine to turn bright yellow (a harmless side effect).

Dietary Sources Include: Dairy products, eggs, green vegetables (including asparagus, romaine lettuce, broccoli, and spinach), mushrooms, meats, Brewer's yeast, and riboflavin-fortified foods and beverages.

Niacin (Nicotinic Acid, Nicotinamide, Niacinamide, Vitamin B₃)

Niacin aids in digestive health and the development and maintenance of nerves and tissues. Like the other B vitamins, it also plays important roles in converting food into energy. It is stable under exposure to heat, light, and air. Tryptophan, an essential amino acid that is one of the building blocks of protein, can be converted to niacin in the body if enough vitamin B_6, riboflavin, and iron are available.[11]

Niacin deficiency is called pellegra, a condition that is very rare in this country due to the existence of niacin-fortified foods. The symptoms of pellagra include what are referred to as the "Four Ds"— dermatitis (skin rash or irritation), diarrhea, dementia (loss of mental functions), and death.

Niacin is associated with a variety of side effects from flushing (reddened skin) to liver toxicity, though they appear to be less prevalent with the nicotinamide (also called niacinimide) form of this nutrient.[12] Taking high doses of supplemental niacin can have serious adverse effects. The UL for adults 19 years of age and older is 35 mg per day including amounts derived from supplements, fortified foods, or both.[13]

---

[11] Higdon, J. and Drake, V.J., Linus Pauling Institute, "Niacin," June 2007, <http://lpi.oregonstate.edu/infocenter/vitamins/niacin/> (March 11, 2009).
[12] See footnote 11.
[13] Institute of Medicine, Food and Nutrition Board, "Zinc," Dietary Reference Intakes for Thiamin, Riboflavin, Niacin, Vitamin B6, Folate, Vitamin B12, Pantothenic Acid, Biotin, and Choline, p. 123. Reprinted with permission from the National Academies Press. Copyright © 1998 National Academy of Sciences.

Dietary Sources Include: Tuna, salmon, chicken, turkey, beef, whole grains, eggs, soy, peanuts, nuts, and niacin-fortified foods and beverages.

Pantothenic Acid (Calcium Pantothenate, Vitamin B_5)

Another of the B complex vitamins involved in the utilization of energy from foods and also an important player in the development of fatty acids, cholesterol, and hormones, pantothenic acid is not only available from many food sources but may also be made by bacteria in our large intestines.[14] Deficiencies of this nutrient are rare. No adverse effects have been associated with high intake.[15] Pantothenic acid is destroyed by exposure to heat, acidity (such as that caused by vinegar), and alkalinity (such as that caused by baking soda).

Dietary Sources Include: Dairy products, fish, shellfish, chicken, beef, liver, eggs, whole grains, wheat germ, broccoli, peas, potatoes, sunflower seeds, legumes, yeast, and pantothenic acid-fortified foods and beverages.

Vitamin B_6 (Pyridoxine)

Vitamin B_6, also known as pyridoxine, is essential for a wide variety of metabolic functions in the body, especially those involved with our nervous and immune systems. In its active coenzyme form as pyridoxal phosphate it is used by more than 100 bodily enzymes that are involved in converting carbohydrates, fats, and proteins into energy.[16] It plays crucial roles in amino

---

[14] Said, H.M., et al., "Biotin uptake by human colonic epithelial NCM460 cells: a carrier-mediated process shared with pantothenic acid," *American Journal of Physiology: Cell Physiology,* November 1998, 275(5Pt1):C1365-1371.

[15] Institute of Medicine, Food and Nutrition Board, "Pantothenic Acid," Dietary Reference Intakes for Thiamin, Riboflavin, Niacin, Vitamin B6, Folate, Vitamin B12, Pantothenic Acid, Biotin, and Choline, p. 370. Reprinted with permission from the National Academies Press. Copyright © 1998 National Academy of Sciences.

[16] Grosvenor, Mary B. and Smolin, Lori A. Nutrition From Science To Life. p. 306. ©2002 Harcourt, Inc. Reproduced with permission of John Wiley and Sons, Inc.

acid metabolism and the regulation of blood sugar and is required for the development of specific neurotransmitters (chemicals that allow nerve cells to communicate with each other).[17] It is also needed for the manufacture of lipids that make up the fatty protective coating on our nerves and the development of both red and white blood cells. Vitamin B_6 is destroyed by exposure to heat, light, and acidic conditions.

Deficiency of this vitamin is relatively rare in the U.S., though the elderly, alcoholics, those who are chronically ill, and those with inadequate diets may be at risk. Deficiency can cause anemia, among other problems. Overconsumption can result in reversible nerve damage of the hands and feet.[18] Vitamin B_6 can cause the urine to turn dark yellow, a harmless side effect.

Dietary Sources Include: Whole grains, lentils, soybeans, eggs, dairy products, potatoes, peas, carrots, spinach, bananas, meat, fish, liver, and vitamin B6-fortified foods and beverages.

Folate (Folic Acid, Vitamin B₉)

Folate, also known as folic acid and vitamin B_9, plays a critical role in the synthesis of our RNA and DNA.[19] It is needed to prevent birth defects that affect the brain and spinal cord. It is also needed to develop red blood cells and prevent a specific type of anemia, as well as to metabolize protein and regulate the level of homocysteine (an amino acid) in the blood.[20] High

[17] Leklem, J.E., "Vitamin B6." In: Shils, M., Olson, J., Shike, M., and Ross, A.C., editors. Modern Nutrition in Health and Disease. 9th ed. Baltimore: Williams & Wilkins, 1999: 413-421. © Lippincott Williams & Wilkins.
[18] National Institutes of Health, "Dietary Supplement Fact Sheet: Vitamin B_6," August 24, 2007, <http://ods.od.nih.gov/factsheets/vitaminb6.asp> (December 13, 2008).
[19] National Institutes of Health, "Dietary Supplement Fact Sheet: Folate," August 22, 2005, <http://dietary-supplements.info.nih.gov/factsheets/folate.asp#h2> (Dec. 13, 2008).
[20] Murphy, Marla, Ohio State University Extension, "Folate (Folacin, Folic Acid)," November 2004, <http://ohioline.osu.edu/hyg-fact/5000/5553.html> (December 13, 2008).

homocysteine levels are associated with a higher risk of coronary heart disease, stroke, and peripheral vascular disease.[21]

In addition to birth defects and anemia, a folate deficiency can cause growth problems. It may also cause a sore tongue, headaches, weakness, heart palpitations, irritability, forgetfulness, and digestive disorders, among other things.[22,23] Alcoholics, those with liver or kidney disease, and those who are pregnant or malnourished are among the individuals most at risk for deficiency.

Although folate is considered to be nontoxic, excess intake can mask anemia caused by a vitamin B_{12} deficiency, which can lead to irreversible nerve damage.[24] It is therefore important to make sure that vitamin B_{12} intake is adequate, and, if anemia is present, to confirm that it is not due to a vitamin B_{12} deficiency. This is especially essential in the elderly.

The folic acid form of folate is usually produced synthetically, as it is rarely found naturally in foods.[25] It is better absorbed by the body than naturally occurring folate.[26] Folate is destroyed when exposed to heat, light, air, and acidity.

Dietary Sources Include: Lentils, whole grains, liver, peas, spinach, asparagus, romaine lettuce, oranges, and folate-fortified foods and beverages.

Vitamin B_{12} (Cobalamin)

Vitamin B_{12} is essential for proper nervous system functioning and the production of blood cells. It also plays important roles in metabolism. Anemia

[21] Source: American Heart Association, "What is Homocysteine?" © 2009 www.americanheart.org.

[22] Herbert, V., "Folic Acid." In: Shils, M., Olson, J., Shike, M., and Ross, A.C., editors. Modern Nutrition in Health and Disease. Baltimore: Williams & Wilkins, 1999: 433-446. © Lippincott Williams & Wilkins.

[23] Haslam, N. and Probert, C.S., "An audit of the investigation and treatment of folic acid deficiency," Journal of the Royal Society of Medicine, 1998, 91:72-3.

[24] National Institutes of Health, "Dietary Supplement Fact Sheet: Folate," n.d., <http://dietary-supplements.info.nih.gov/factsheets/folate.asp#h9> (December 12, 2008).

[25] Grosvenor, Mary B. and Smolin, Lori A. Nutrition From Science To Life. p. 310. ©2002 Harcourt, Inc. Reproduced with permission of John Wiley and Sons, Inc.

[26] See footnote 24.

that results from a deficiency of this vitamin may be masked by high consumption of folic acid.[27] Vegans and other vegetarians may need to take it as a supplement if sufficient amounts are not consumed in the diet. Those at risk for deficiency include alcoholics, the elderly, and individuals with ulcers or other gastrointestinal disorders. Vitamin B_{12} is destroyed by exposure to light and air. There is no known toxicity to this vitamin.

Dietary Sources Include: Meats, dairy products, eggs, shellfish, and vitamin B_{12}-fortified foods and beverages.

___

Biotin

Like most of the other B vitamins, biotin is important in the utilization of energy from foods. It is also essential in the metabolism of cholesterol as well as the metabolism of certain fatty acids and amino acids.[28] Deficiencies are very rare, though when they do occur they can cause hair loss, facial and genital rashes, depression, lethargy, hallucinations, and tingling and numbness in the extremities, among other effects.[29] There is no known toxicity to this nutrient. A protein in raw egg whites called avidin binds biotin, thereby rendering it unavailable for absorption by the body (one more reason not to eat raw cookie dough made with eggs). Biotin is destroyed by exposure to heat.

Dietary Sources Include: Liver, eggs, yeast, wheat bran, whole grains, nuts, yogurt, broccoli, legumes, avocados, and biotin-fortified foods and beverages.

___

[27] Grosvenor, Mary B. and Smolin, Lori A. Nutrition From Science To Life. p. 317. © 2002 Harcourt, Inc. Reproduced with permission of John Wiley and Sons, Inc.
[28] Zempleni J. and Mock, D.M., "Biotin biochemistry and human requirements," *Journal of Nutritional Biochemistry,* 1999; 10:128-138. Copyright © 1999 Elsevier Science Inc. Reprinted with permission from Elsevier.
[29] Higdon, J. and Drake, V.J., Linus Pauling Institute, "Biotin," August 2008, <http://lpi.oregonstate.edu/infocenter/vitamins/biotin/index.html> (December 13, 2008).

Choline

While not an actual vitamin but rather an essential nutrient often grouped with the B vitamins, choline is needed for a variety of different functions in the body including cell communication, muscle control, memory, and the metabolism of fats.[30] High intake (more than 10 grams per day) can have toxic effects. Those who avoid milk and eggs (including vegans and those with allergies, sensitivities, or aversions to these foods) may be at risk for choline deficiency. The Food and Nutrition Board of the National Academy of Sciences recommends 550 mg of choline daily for adult men and 425 mg daily for adult women.

Dietary Sources Include: Wheat germ, eggs, beef liver, beef, broccoli, shrimp, salmon, cod, peanut butter, milk, milk chocolate, and choline-fortified foods and beverages.[31]

Vitamin C (Ascorbate, Ascorbic Acid)

Vitamin C is a water-soluble antioxidant vitamin that helps to bolster the immune system and is essential for healing. It is needed to form collagen, a strong, fibrous protein found in many parts of the body including the skin, bones, teeth, muscles, heart, and blood vessels. It aids in the absorption of non-heme iron (a form of iron found mainly in many plant-based foods) and is needed for the development of specific neurotransmitters (chemicals essential to brain function) and hormones. It also assists in the body's development of carnitine, an amino acid-derived compound that assists in turning fat into energy.[32] A highly fragile nutrient, it is destroyed by air,

[30] Higdon, J. and Drake, V.J., Linus Pauling Institute, "Choline," January 2008, <http://lpi.oregonstate.edu/infocenter/othernuts/choline/> (December 13, 2008).
[31] U.S. Department of Agriculture, USDA Database for the Choline Content of Common Foods–2004, <http://www.nal.usda.gov/fnic/foodcomp/Data/Choline/Choline.html>.
[32] Carr, A.C. and Frei, B., "Toward a new recommended dietary allowance for vitamin C based on antioxidant and health effects in humans," *American Journal of Clinical Nutrition,* June 1999;69(6):1086-1107.

heat, and light as well as contact with iron and can also be lost when foods are boiled or steamed.

A lack of vitamin C in the body can cause scurvy, which is characterized by a number of symptoms including dry hair and skin, inflamed or bleeding gums, slow wound healing, easy bruising, nosebleeds, sore joints, and anemia. Scurvy is rare, though it is a risk factor for alcoholics and those who are malnourished or consume little or no fruits and vegetables.

Overconsumption of vitamin C, on the other hand, can cause abdominal cramps, nausea, and diarrhea among those in good health, and may cause additional symptoms among those whose health is compromised. In addition, while consuming too little vitamin C can affect the integrity of both teeth and gums, excess consumption of chewable or powdered forms of this nutrient can lead to tooth erosion.[33]

Vitamin C's overall role in the prevention and treatment of disease is still under investigation. While one study suggested that vitamin C may damage DNA and enhance the potential for cancer, it failed to take several factors into consideration that involve the chemistry of the human body.[34]

Many other studies have actually shown that the use of vitamin C is associated with *decreased* incidence of cancers of the bladder, cervix, colon-rectum, esophagus, lungs, pancreas, salivary glands, stomach, throat, and vocal cords.[35,36] Research has also shown that consumption of vitamin C can reduce the duration of the common cold.[37] Obtaining this vitamin from food appears to be best.

---

[33] Ali, D.A., Brown, R.S., Rodriguez, L.O., Moody, E.L., and Nasr, M.F., "Dental erosion caused by silent gastroesophageal reflux disease," *JADA,* 2002; 133(6):734-37.Copyright © 2002 American Dental Association. All rights reserved. Adapted 2009 with permission.

[34] Frei, Balz, "Vitamin C Doesn't Cause Cancer!" November 2001, <http://lpi.oregonstate.edu/f-w01/cancer.html> (December 13, 2008).

[35] Higdon, J., "Vitamin C," Linus Pauling Institute, January 2006, <http://lpi.oregonstate.edu/infocenter/vitamins/vitaminC/> (December 13, 2006).

[36] Head, K.A., "Ascorbic acid in the prevention and treatment of cancer," *Alternative Medicine Review,* June 1998, 3(3):174-86.

[37] Douglas, R.M. and Hemilä, H. "Vitamin C for Preventing and Treating the Common Cold," *PLoS Medicine,* June 28, 2005, 2(6): e168.

Dietary Sources Include: Citrus fruits, strawberries, raspberries, blueberries, cranberries, mango, pineapple, cantaloupe, tomatoes, red and green bell peppers, broccoli, snow peas, potatoes, and vitamin C-fortified foods and beverages. All fruits and vegetables contain vitamin C in varying amounts.

Fat-Soluble Vitamins

Vitamin A (Retinol)
Vitamin A, also called retinol due to its vision-promoting properties involving the eye's retina, is needed for the formation and maintenance of teeth, bones, skin, hair, and mucous membranes; the development, functioning, and regulation of cells; and the prevention and treatment of night blindness. It is essential for growth, reproduction, and proper functioning of the immune system.

Vitamin A exists both preformed (ready to be utilized by the body) and as a precursor or "provitamin" (a substance that is converted to an active vitamin in the body). Each type is found in the diet as well as in nutritional supplement form. Preformed sources of vitamin A are called retinoids, which include retinal, retinol, and retinoic acid. Precursor sources are called carotenoids. The most common carotenoid is beta carotene, an antioxidant which is found naturally in red, orange, and yellow fruits and vegetables. Synthetically produced beta carotene is often added to processed foods such as margarine and cheese. Preformed vitamin A, which is generally found in higher amounts in supplements rather than foods, does not need to be converted in the body and can be toxic when eaten in quantities higher than the UL established by the Food and Nutrition Board of the National Academy of Sciences. For infants and children up to three years of age this amount should not exceed 600 µg (micrograms) per day; children four to eight years of age 900 µg per day; males and females nine to thirteen years of age 1,700 µg per day; males and females fourteen to eighteen years of age 2,800 µg per day; and males and females nineteen to seventy years of age 3,000 µg per day. Both vitamin A and beta carotene are destroyed by exposure to light, air, and acidic conditions. Beta carotene may turn the urine deep yellow or orange.

Dietary Sources Include: Liver, eggs, butter, sweet potatoes, carrots, pumpkin, turnip greens, spinach, papaya, mangos, apricots, cantaloupe, and vitamin A-fortified foods and beverages, including milk.

Vitamin D
Vitamin D, which is often referred to as "vitamin D hormone" by scientists due to the fact that its structure and activity closely resemble that of a hormone, exists in two forms: as vitamin D_3 (also called cholecalciferol) and as vitamin D_2 (also called ergocalciferol). Vitamin D_3 is the natural form of vitamin D. It is found in some fish and animal-based foods and is also produced when our skin is exposed to ultraviolet light such as sunlight (gaining it the nickname "the Sunshine Vitamin"). Vitamin D_2, on the other hand, is synthetically produced.

Vitamin D's primary role in the body is to maintain normal levels of the minerals calcium and phosphorus in the bloodstream by aiding in their absorption. This is essential for the development and maintenance of teeth and bones.

Vitamin D consumed in naturally occurring foods does not cause toxicity, nor does vitamin D that is produced when the skin is exposed to sunlight.[38] Vitamin D taken in supplement form or consumed in fortified foods, however, can cause toxicity when taken in amounts higher than the established UL (50 µg daily for adults 19 years of age and older).

A deficiency of vitamin D can lead to rickets in children and osteomalacia in adults, two diseases associated with bone deformity. Those at risk for deficiency include children, breastfed infants, the elderly, extreme dieters, and individuals with kidney disease or gastrointestinal disorders.

[38] Grosvenor, Mary B. and Smolin, Lori A. <u>Nutrition From Science To Life</u>. p. 339. ©2002 Harcourt, Inc. Reproduced with permission of John Wiley and Sons, Inc.

Vitamin D is destroyed when exposed to air, light, heat, and conditions that lack sufficient acidity.

Dietary Sources Include: Cod liver oil, salmon, mackerel, sardines, tuna, eggs, cheese, margarine, beef liver, and vitamin D-fortified foods and beverages, including milk.

Vitamin E

Like vitamins A and C, vitamin E is an antioxidant (a substance that helps to prevent the damaging effects of unstable molecules known as free radicals). It is important in reproduction and the protection of cell membranes, which it can defend from damage by heavy metals, toxins, drugs, and environmental pollutants. [39]

Vitamin E exists in eight different forms. The form that is most active in the human body is alpha-tocopherol.[40] Synthetic alpha-tocopherol (which begins with the prefix "dl" as in dl-alpha tocopherol) is not absorbed by the body as effectively as natural alpha-tocopherol (which begins with the prefix "d" as in d-alpha tocopherol). Both vitamin E deficiency and toxicity are rare, though supplemental doses above the recommended UL may interfere with vitamin K's blood clotting effects and increase the possibility of hemorrhage. This is an especially important consideration for those taking blood thinners.

Vitamin E is destroyed by exposure to light, air, and extreme hot and cold temperatures.

Dietary Sources Include: Wheat germ oil, sunflower oil, safflower oil, sunflower seeds, almonds, hazelnuts, peanut butter, olives, sweet potatoes, avocados, and vitamin E-fortified foods and beverages.

---

[39] Grosvenor, Mary B. and Smolin, Lori A. Nutrition From Science To Life. p. 347. ©2002 Harcourt, Inc. Reproduced with permission of John Wiley and Sons, Inc.
[40] National Institutes of Health, "Vitamin E," January 23, 2007, <http://dietary-supplements.info.nih.gov/factsheets/vitamine.asp#h5> (December 13, 2008).

Vitamin K (Phylloquinone, Menaquinones)

Vitamin K is essential for blood clotting. It exists in several forms and is found in both plant- and animal-based foods. Phylloquinone (also previously called vitamin K_1) is the plant form of vitamin K. Menaquinones (previously called vitamin K_2) are a group of animal-based forms of vitamin K, which include those that can be made in the body from normal bacteria in our intestines.

Vitamin K deficiency is rare, though gastrointestinal disorders are a risk factor. Natural vitamin K has no known toxicity, although it can interfere with the action of anticoagulant drugs. Vitamin K is destroyed by exposure to light.

Dietary Sources Include: Soybeans, peas, cauliflower, cabbage, green leafy vegetables, liver, olive oil, canola oil, milk chocolate, and vitamin K-fortified foods and beverages.

Minerals

Like vitamins, minerals are micronutrients. Unlike vitamins, they are not destroyed by exposure to heat or air, or by acid or alkaline conditions, though they can be lost from foods during refinement (such as when whole wheat is made into refined white flour), preparation (such as when fruits and vegetables are peeled), and cooking (such as when potatoes are boiled and lose their water-soluble potassium). They are found in both plant- and animal-based foods as well as in fish and seafood. They are also found in a variety of supplemental forms, including as liquids, chewables, and tablets. There are two basic types: major minerals (also called macrominerals) and trace minerals (also called trace elements or microminerals). Major minerals need to be acquired in the diet in amounts greater than 100 mg (milligrams) daily, while trace minerals are required in daily amounts of 100 mg or less.

Minerals are essential for the regulation of chemical and cellular processes in the body. They also play critical roles in the development and maintenance of the body's structural parts. For example, calcium is needed for the secretion of certain hormones; iron is needed for the development of hemoglobin in red blood cells; and calcium, magnesium, and phosphorus are required for healthy bones.

Like other nutrients, the amount of minerals found in foods and beverages (including water) can vary greatly. In addition, the amount of each mineral that is effectively absorbed by the body (known as its bioavailability) can vary due to a variety of factors including age, health, and dietary considerations.

Here is a closer look at the various types of minerals in the diet along with some of the foods they are found in:

Major Minerals (Macrominerals)

Calcium
Calcium is the most prevalent mineral in the body. The majority of this nutrient (about 99%) is found in our teeth and bones; the rest is found in our blood and muscles and in the fluid between our cells.[41,42] It is essential for growth and maintenance as well as a variety of other vital bodily functions. It works together with magnesium, phosphorus, and vitamin D. Consistently maintaining adequate levels of calcium throughout life is an important factor in preventing osteoporosis.

When calcium is consumed with lactose (a natural sugar found in milk and milk products), its absorption is increased; when it is consumed with oxalates, fiber, tannins, or phytate, its absorption is decreased (though when overall calcium intake is adequate these inhibiting factors have little effect on the body's calcium status).[43] Oxalates are compounds found in a wide variety of foods including spinach, whole wheat, blueberries, chocolate, and

[41] Weaver, C.M. and Heaney, R.P., "Calcium." In: Shils, M., Shike, M., Ross, A.C., Caballero, B., and Cousins, R.J., editors. Modern Nutrition in Health and Disease. Tenth edition. Baltimore: Lippincott Williams & Wilkins, 2005:196. Copyright © Lippincott Williams & Wilkins.

[42] National Institutes of Health, "Calcium," December 4, 2008, <http://ods.od.nih.gov/factsheets/calcium.asp#en1> (December 13, 2008).

[43] Grosvenor, Mary B. and Smolin, Lori A. Nutrition From Science To Life. p. 411. © 2002 Harcourt, Inc. Reproduced with permission of John Wiley and Sons, Inc.

soy (for a more complete list visit **http://patient education.upmc.com/ Pdf/Low OxalateDiet.pdf**). Fiber is found predominantly in lentils, beans, peas, and whole grains. Tannins are found in numerous foods and beverages including red wine, tea, chocolate, bananas, betel nuts, and cow-peas. Phytate is found in whole grains, beans, nuts, and sesame seeds, among other foods. Some foods that are high in oxalates, fiber, tannins, or phytate (or a combination of these) are also high in calcium, which may help to offset their effect on calcium absorption.

High consumption of alcohol, sodium, or protein can also affect calcium levels in the body. Excessive intake of alcohol causes the body to lose calcium, and excessive intake of sodium or protein can cause the body to lose additional calcium when the amount of calcium being consumed is already insufficient.[44]

Calcium absorption is also affected by our age and the amount of vitamin D we consume. As we age, we absorb less than half the amount of calcium we absorbed during infancy (pregnancy is an exception, as the body absorbs more calcium during this time with the help of estrogen).[45] A deficiency of vitamin D can further reduce absorption.

Consuming too much calcium also has negative effects. Studies have shown that high dietary calcium intake is associated with impaired kidney function, a reduction in the absorption of zinc and other minerals, and elevated levels of calcium in the blood (a rare condition).[46,47] The body can only effectively utilize approximately 500 mg of calcium at one time.[48]

---

[44] National Institutes of Health, NIAMS, "Calcium and Vitamin D: Important at Every Age," *Nutrition and Bone Health,* January 2009, < http://www.niams.nih.gov/Health_Info/ Bone/Bone_Health/Nutrition/default.asp> (April 2, 2009).

[45] See footnote 43.

[46] Wood, R.J. and Zheng, J.J., "High dietary calcium intakes reduce zinc absorption and balance in humans," *American Journal of Clinical Nutrition,* 1997; 65:1803-1809, <http://www.ajcn.org/cgi/content/abstract/65/6/1803> (December 13, 2008).

[47] Standing Committee on the Scientific Evaluation of Dietary Reference Intakes, Food and Nutrition Board, Institute of Medicine. Dietary Reference Intakes for Calcium, Phosphorus, Magnesium, Vitamin D and Fluoride, p. 140. Reprinted with permission from the National Academies Press. Copyright © 1997 National Academy of Sciences.

[48] See footnote 44.

In supplement form, calcium citrate has been shown to be more bio-available than calcium carbonate.[49] It may also be better absorbed by the elderly and others who have lower levels of stomach acid. Microcrystalline calcium hydroxyapatite has also been found to be an excellent bioavailable form of calcium.[50]

Dietary Sources Include: Milk, cream, yogurt, cheese, almonds, spinach, broccoli, kale, salmon (canned, with bones) and calcium-fortified foods and beverages.

Sodium (Sodium Chloride)

Sodium, also commonly known as sodium chloride or table salt, acts both as a mineral and an electrolyte (an electrolyte is an element found in bodily fluids that is necessary for cellular, muscular, and nerve-related functions, among other things). Excess consumption of sodium can lead to hypertension (high blood pressure) and other health problems. The USDA's Dietary Guidelines for Americans recommends that Americans consume less than 2,300 mg (about one teaspoon) of sodium daily along with potassium-rich fruits and vegetables, and that individuals with hypertension, blacks, and middle-aged and older adults aim to consume no more than 1,500 mg of sodium per day while meeting the potassium recommendation of 4,700 mg per day from foods at the same time.

It has been estimated that only a little over one tenth of the sodium in the average American diet is found naturally in foods, and that nearly eighty percent is added during food processing.[51] It is often found in processed

---

[49] Heller, H.J., et al., "Pharmacokinetic and pharmacodynamic comparison of two calcium supplements in postmenopausal women," *Journal of Clinical Pharm.*, 40:1237-1244. Copyright © 2000 American College of Clinical Pharmacology, Inc. Reprinted by Permission of SAGE Publications.

[50] Windsor, A.C.M., et al., "The effect of whole-bone extract on [47]Ca absorption in the elderly," *Age and Ageing,* November 1973; 2:230-4. Copyright © 1973 British Geriatrics Society. Reprinted with permission from Oxford University Press.

[51] Mattes, R.D. and Donnelly, D, "Relative contributions of dietary sodium sources," *Journal of the American College of Nutrition,* August 1991, 10(4):383-93.

foods in the form of sodium citrate, sodium glutamate, and sodium bicarbonate (baking soda). Sodium deficiency is rare.

Dietary Sources Include: Virtually all foods and many beverages except those that are specifically labeled as being sodium free. Higher-salt foods and beverages include many soups, pizzas, and snack foods as well as salt-added tomato and vegetable juices. Lower-sodium foods include fresh fruits and vegetables, whole grains, unsalted butter, unsalted or low-salt nuts and nut butters, eggs, unsalted popcorn, and many dairy products.

Chloride

Similar to sodium (and also potassium), chloride is both a mineral and an electrolyte. It works together with sodium and bicarbonate to regulate the body's acid-base balance. It is a major component of both table salt (in the form of sodium chloride) and some salt substitutes (in the form of potassium chloride) in addition to being found in a variety of natural foods. Deficiency is uncommon. Toxicity has only been reported in remote cases of impaired sodium chloride metabolism.

Dietary Sources Include: Table salt, tomatoes, celery, olives, rye, kelp, and chloride-fortified foods and beverages, including some bottled waters.

Potassium

Like sodium and chloride, potassium has vital dual roles as both a mineral and an electrolyte and helps regulate the body's acid-base balance. It is necessary not only for cellular communication in the body, but also for kidney, heart, muscle, bone, and digestive tract health.[52] It works together with sodium to conduct nerve impulses in the body. Unlike sodium and chloride, it

---

[52] Higdon, J. and Drake, V., Linus Pauling Institute, "Potassium," November 2007, <http://lpi.oregonstate.edu/infocenter/minerals/potassium/> (December 13, 2008).

is generally found in higher amounts in unprocessed natural foods (e.g., bananas, potatoes) than in those that are processed.

Both deficiency and high blood levels of potassium can have serious effects on health. A deficiency, called hypokalemia, can cause a variety of symptoms including fatigue, gastrointestinal problems (e.g., intestinal paralysis) and weakness and cramping of the muscles.[53] It can also cause irregular heartbeat especially (and ironically) in those taking diuretics to *treat* high blood pressure or heart disease.[54,55] Vomiting, diarrhea, rare kidney and adrenal gland diseases, extreme dieting without nutritional support, extended fasts, and the use of laxatives can also cause potassium deficiency.

High blood levels of potassium, known as hyperkalemia, are also a concern. They are rarely due to overconsumption, but rather tend to occur when kidney function is poor and potassium intake is normal or high, or when potassium-sparing drugs such as diuretics are being taken.[56]

Dietary Sources Include: Bananas, cantaloupe, citrus fruits, prunes, raisins, tomatoes, potatoes, legumes, spinach, broccoli, winter squash, beet greens, Swiss chard, red meat, chicken, salmon, sardines, molasses, and potassium-fortified foods and beverages including milks and yogurts.

Magnesium

Magnesium is needed to maintain normal functioning of the muscles, nerves, heart, and immune system and is essential to good bone health. It also helps regulate blood sugar levels, is necessary for turning fats, carbohydrates, and protein into energy, and promotes normal blood pressure by affecting how

---

[53] See footnote 52.

[54] Panel on Dietary Reference Intakes for Electrolytes and Water, Standing Committee on the Scientific Evaluation of Dietary Reference Intakes, "Potassium," Dietary Reference Intakes for Water, Potassium, Sodium, Chloride, and Sulfate, pp. 186-188. Reprinted with permission from the National Academies Press. Copyright © 2004 National Academy of Sciences.

[55] Gennari, F.J., "Hypokalemia," *New England Journal of Medicine,* August 13, 1998, 339(7): 451-458.

[56] See footnote 52.

the electrolytes calcium, potassium, and sodium are metabolized.[57],[58] Overall it is needed for more than 300 biochemical reactions in the body.[59] It works well together with calcium.

Alcoholics, those with severely restricted or inadequate diets, those on diuretics, diabetics, and those with kidney disease or gastrointestinal disorders are among the individuals at risk for deficiency of this nutrient. Deficiency has been linked to severity and frequency of migraine headaches, some forms of heart attacks, high blood pressure, sleep disorders, and mood disturbances.[60] Toxicity is uncommon and unlikely to result from food intake, however it can occur from the overuse of supplements or drugs that contain magnesium, including various laxatives and antacids.

Dietary Sources Include: Wheat germ, oat bran, brown rice, nuts, seeds, beans, peas, bananas, kiwi, spinach, Swiss chard, blackstrap molasses, and magnesium-fortified foods and beverages. Hard water (water that is high in minerals) can also contain magnesium, often in substantial amounts.

Phosphorus
Phosphorus plays important roles in bone, tooth, and cell structure and is essential to the development of both our DNA and RNA. It is also required for the production, storage, and disbursement of energy, the regulation of hormones and enzymes, the balance of pH in cells, and many other important metabolic functions.

Deficiencies of phosphorus are rare, though premature infants, vegans, alcoholics, the elderly, those on extended fasts, and those with chronic

[57] Wester, P.O., "Magnesium," *American Journal of Clinical Nutrition,* 1987, 45:1305-12.
[58] Saris, N.E., et al., "Magnesium: an update on physiological, clinical, and analytical aspects," *Clinica Chimica Acta,* April 2000, 294:1-26. Copyright © 2000 Elsevier Science B.V. Reprinted with permission from Elsevier.
[59] National Institutes of Health, "Magnesium," December 5, 2005, <http://ods.od.nih.gov/factsheets/magnesium.asp>. (December 13, 2008).
[60] Neilsen, Forrest H., "Migraines, Sleeplessness, Heart Attacks—Magnesium?" October 23, 2006, <http://www.ars.usda.gov/News/docs.htm?docid=10874> (December 13, 2008).

vomiting or diarrhea are at risk. Those who repeatedly consume antacids that contain calcium, aluminum, or magnesium are also at risk.[61]

Dietary Sources Include: Whole grains, dairy products, apples, apricots, oranges, asparagus, broccoli, beans, nuts, seeds, meats, sardines, and phosphorus-fortified foods and beverages.

Sulfur

Sulfur is needed in the body for the development of protein, the detoxification of drugs, and the protection of cells from oxidative damage, as well as for regulation of the body's acid-base balance.[62] Although it may also be useful in treating allergies, pain, depression, diabetes, cancer, AIDS, and other health conditions, its effects on human health have not been extensively studied.

Deficiency is rare, though it has the potential to occur when protein needs are unmet, such as during extreme dieting or in cases of malnutrition. Children, vegan athletes, and those who are HIV-positive are also at risk.[63] The risk of toxicity from foods is low.

Dietary Sources Include: Protein-based foods and beverages, as well as those that contain sulfur dioxide, sodium sulfite, sodium bisulfite, or potassium bisulfite as preservatives. Thiamin (vitamin B_1) and biotin also contain sulfur.

---

[61] Evidence-based Systematic Review of Phosphates, Phosphorus by the Natural Standard Research Collaboration. Natural Standard (www.naturalstandard.com) last accessed 12/13/08. Copyright©2009. Somerville, MA USA.

[62] Grosvenor, Mary B. and Smolin, Lori A. Nutrition From Science To Life. p. 429. ©2002 Harcourt, Inc. Reproduced with permission of John Wiley and Sons, Inc.

[63] Parcell, Stephen, "Sulfur in Human Nutrition and Applications in Medicine," *Alternative Medicine Review,* February 2002, 7(1):22-44, <http://www.thorne.com/media/sulfur.pdf>.

Trace Minerals (Microminerals)

Iron

Iron is needed to deliver oxygen to cells and remove carbon dioxide from the body. It is also essential for growth and development, energy production, drug metabolism, protection from oxidative damage, and efficient functioning of the immune system.[64] It is found in both plant- and animal-based foods. There are two types: heme and nonheme. Heme iron is found exclusively in animal-based foods, while nonheme iron is found mainly in foods that are derived from plants. Of the two, heme iron is more readily absorbed by the body.[65] Iron supplements, which are derived from nonheme iron, are available in two forms: ferric and ferrous. The ferrous form, which is available as iron salts including ferrous gluconate, ferrous fumarate, and ferrous sulfate, is absorbed best by the body.[66]

As with calcium, the body's absorption of nonheme iron can be inhibited by fiber, phytate, tannins, and oxalates. Other minerals and certain vegetable proteins (including soy protein) may also inhibit absorption.[67] Absorption can be increased by consuming a source of heme iron together with a source of nonheme iron, such as by eating a meal that contains both meat and beans. Absorption can also be increased by amino acids, sugars, and vitamin C.[68] It is important to eat a balanced diet that includes iron-containing foods, as only 1 mg of iron is absorbed for every 10 to 20 mg of iron ingested.[69]

---

[64] Grosvenor, Mary B. and Smolin, Lori A. Nutrition From Science To Life. p. 436. ©2002 Harcourt, Inc. Reproduced with permission of John Wiley and Sons, Inc.

[65] Miret S., Simpson, R.J., and McKie, A.T., " Physiology and molecular biology of dietary iron absorption." Reprinted with permission from the Annual Review of Nutrition, Volume 23, ©2003 by Annual Reviews. www.annualreviews.org.

[66] National Anemia Action Council, "A Patient's Guide to Oral Iron Supplements," November 14, 2008, <http://www.anemia.org/patients/feature-articles/content.php?contentid=000316>.

[67] Grosvenor, Mary B. and Smolin, Lori A. Nutrition From Science To Life. p. 435. ©2002 Harcourt, Inc. Reproduced with permission of John Wiley and Sons, Inc.

[68] Grosvenor, Mary B. and Smolin, Lori A. Nutrition From Science To Life. p. 434. ©2002 Harcourt, Inc. Reproduced with permission of John Wiley and Sons, Inc.

[69] University of Maryland Medical Center, "Iron-Deficiency Anemia," January 30, 2008, <http://www.umm.edu/blood/aneiron.htm> (December 13, 2008).

Iron deficiency causes anemia. It is the most common nutritional deficiency in this country.[70] Overconsumption is also a concern. Taking too much iron in supplement form can cause toxicity (which can be life threatening) and interfere with the body's absorption of both zinc and copper.[71] Toxicity can be acute (resulting from a single large dose of supplemental iron) or chronic (due to a slow accumulation of iron from foods or supplements over time). Chronic toxicity, commonly referred to as iron overload, is most commonly caused by a genetic disorder known as hereditary hemochromatosis (also called primary hemochromatosis), though it can also be due to anemia, alcoholism, and other disorders (in these latter causes it is referred to as secondary hemochromatosis).[72] Iron works together with vitamin B_{12} and folate.

Dietary Sources Include: Lentils, peas, spinach, liver, beef, poultry, shellfish, salmon, whole grains, sunflower seeds, parsley, and iron-fortified foods and beverages. Nonheme iron also leaches from iron cookware and utensils into foods (especially acidic foods such as tomatoes).

Zinc

Of all the trace minerals found within the body's cells, zinc is the most abundant.[73] It is necessary for the functioning of more than 300 different enzymes and plays a vital role in numerous biological processes including bone and tissue development, immune system activity, the regulation of insulin, and the conversion of thyroid hormones.[74] It is also a cofactor for

[70] Centers for Disease Control and Prevention, "Recommendations to Prevent and Control Iron Deficiency in the United States," <http://www.cdc.gov/mmwr/preview/mmwrhtml/00051880.htm> (December 13, 2008).
[71] Grosvenor, Mary B. and Smolin, Lori A. Nutrition From Science To Life. p. 442. ©2002 Harcourt, Inc. Reproduced with permission of John Wiley and Sons, Inc.
[72] National Institutes of Health, "Hemochromatosis," *Publication No 07-4621,* April 2007, <http://digestive.niddk.nih.gov/ddiseases/pubs/hemochromatosis/index.htm>.
[73] Grosvenor, Mary B. and Smolin, Lori A. Nutrition From Science To Life. p. 446. ©2002 Harcourt, Inc. Reproduced with permission of John Wiley and Sons, Inc.
[74] Evidence-based Systematic Review of Zinc by the Natural Standard Research Collaboration. Natural Standard (www.naturalstandard.com) last accessed 12/13/08. Copyright©2009. Somerville, MA USA.

one form of the antioxidant enzyme known as superoxide dismutase (SOD), and is an important player in a number of enzymatic reactions involving carbohydrate and protein metabolism.[75,76] It is found in both plant- and animal-based foods, though it is better absorbed from those that are animal-based due to the fact that they do not contain phytate.[77]

Zinc deficiency can result in a wide array of health problems including poor growth, hair loss, skin conditions, impotence, and decreased immunity.[78,79] At risk are those who are malnourished, alcoholic, or have a genetic defect in zinc absorption and metabolism (a condition known as acrodermatitis enteropathica); those who consume low-protein, high-phytate diets; and those who have chronic diseases such as sickle-cell anemia, kidney disease, cancer, or AIDS.[80]

Zinc toxicity is also a concern. Large doses taken by mouth even for a short time can cause stomach cramps, nausea, and vomiting; taken longer, they can cause anemia and decrease the levels of our good cholesterol.[81] Consuming foods or beverages from galvanized containers raises the risk of zinc toxicity. The National Academies of Sciences' UL for zinc for adults is 40 mg per day from all sources.[82]

---

[75] See footnote 73.

[76] See footnote 74.

[77] Grosvenor, Mary B. and Smolin, Lori A. Nutrition From Science To Life. p. 407. ©2002 Harcourt, Inc. Reproduced with permission of John Wiley and Sons, Inc.

[78] "Zinc," Dietary Reference Intakes for Vitamin A, Vitamin K, Arsenic, Boron, Chromium, Copper, Iodine, Iron, Manganese, Molybdenum, Nickel, Silicon, Vanadium, and Zinc. p. 447. Reprinted with permission from the National Academies Press. Copyright © 2000 National Academy of Sciences.

[79]Shankar, A.H., and Prasad, A.S., " Zinc and immune function: the biological basis of altered resistance to infection," American Journal of Clinical Nutrition, 1998 Aug; 68 (2 Suppl): 447S-463S.

[80] Grosvenor, Mary B. and Smolin, Lori A. Nutrition From Science To Life. p. 447. ©2002 Harcourt, Inc. Reproduced with permission of John Wiley and Sons, Inc.

[81] Centers for Disease Control and Prevention, ToxFAQs™ for Zinc, August 2005, <http://www.atsdr.cdc.gov/tfacts60.pdf> (March 11, 2009).

[82] "Zinc," Dietary Reference Intakes for Vitamin A, Vitamin K, Arsenic, Boron, Chromium, Copper, Iodine, Iron, Manganese, Molybdenum, Nickel, Silicon, Vanadium, and Zinc. p. 442. Reprinted with permission from the National Academies Press. Copyright © 2000 National Academy of Sciences.

Zinc works together with natural folate to aid in folate absorption and is necessary for the transport and functioning of vitamins A and D.[83] It may interact with herbs and supplements that contain caffeine or have blood pressure-altering, antibiotic, hormonal, diabetic, hypoglycemic, or diuretic effects.[84] For a detailed description of potential herb, supplement, and drug interactions related to zinc visit **www.nlm.nih.gov/medlineplus/druginfo/ natural/ patient-zinc.html.**

Dietary Sources Include: Red meat, poultry, pork, liver, crabmeat, oysters (an extremely good source), whole grains, dairy products, eggs, beans, nuts, seeds, and zinc-fortified foods and beverages.

Copper

Copper is necessary for heart health as well as for the metabolism of iron and lipids, the development of connective tissue, and proper functioning of our immune and central nervous systems.[85] It is also needed for blood clotting, the development of brain chemicals, and the metabolism of both glucose and cholesterol. It may be useful in the treatment of certain cases of iron deficiency anemia.

Copper absorption can be hindered by consuming high levels of iron, manganese, molybdenum, and zinc, in particular. Vitamin C also decreases copper absorption, as can the overuse of antacids.[86,87] In addition to dietary considerations, rare genetic diseases (Wilson's disease, Menkes disease) affect the body's ability to utilize copper.

[83] Grosvenor, Mary B. and Smolin, Lori A. Nutrition From Science To Life. pp. 446-447. © 2002 Harcourt, Inc. Reproduced with permission of John Wiley and Sons, Inc.
[84] Evidence-based Systematic Review of Zinc by the Natural Standard Research Collaboration. Natural Standard (www.naturalstandard.com) last accessed 12/13/08. Copyright©2009. Somerville, MA USA.
[85] Uauy, R., Olivares, M., and Gonzales, M., "Essentiality of copper in humans," American Journal of Clinical Nutrition 1998, 67: 952S-959S.
[86] Wapnir, R.A., "Copper absorption and availability," American Journal of Clinical Nutrition, 1998, 67: 1054S-1060S.
[87] Grosvenor, Mary B. and Smolin, Lori A. Nutrition From Science To Life. p. 448. ©2002 Harcourt, Inc. Reproduced with permission of John Wiley and Sons, Inc.

Overconsumption of copper is toxic. Toxicity is rare, though consuming acidic foods or beverages stored in copper containers poses a risk.

Dietary Sources Include: Shrimp, oysters, lobster, whole grains, beans, nuts, seeds, oat bran, liver, potatoes, spinach, cocoa, chocolate, and copper-fortified foods and beverages.

Manganese

Manganese activates a number of important enzymes in the body and is a building block of others. It is instrumental in a variety of bodily functions and activities including the development of cartilage, the development and functioning of antioxidants, and the metabolism of carbohydrates, cholesterol, and amino acids.[88]

Manganese deficiency is unlikely due to the wide range of foods that contain it. Excess consumption is of more concern, as it can lead to toxicity and result in what is known as "manganese madness," a disorder characterized by an initial onset of mental symptoms including mood swings, compulsiveness, nervousness, irritability, hallucinations, delusions, and unaccountable laughter.

Iron, magnesium, and calcium may affect the bioavailability of this important nutrient.[89]

Dietary Sources Include: Whole grains, legumes, nuts, tea, fruits, vegetables, and manganese-fortified foods and beverages.

---

[88] "Manganese," Dietary Reference Intakes for Vitamin A, Vitamin K, Arsenic, Boron, Chromium, Copper, Iodine, Iron, Manganese, Molybdenum, Nickel, Silicon, Vanadium, and Zinc,
p. 394. Reprinted with permission from the National Academies Press. Copyright © 2000 National Academy of Sciences.
[89] Higdon, J., and Drake, V., Linus Pauling Institute, "Manganese," June 2007,
<http://lpi.oregonstate.edu/infocenter/minerals/manganese/> (December13, 2008).

Selenium

Selenium is needed for proper thyroid and immune system health as well as for the protection of cells from oxidative damage caused by free radicals. It also protects the body against the toxic effects of cadmium and mercury.[90]

Studies have shown that selenium is likely to play an important role in cancer prevention.[91] However, studies have also shown that supplemental selenium may cause diabetes.[92]

In the U.S. both deficiency and toxicity of this trace mineral are rare.

For a detailed overview of selenium visit **http://ods.od.nih.gov/fact sheets/selenium.asp#h4**.

Dietary Sources Include: Brazil nuts (may contain high levels), tuna, crab, salmon, turkey, chicken, beef, eggs, oats, sunflower seeds, and selenium-fortified foods and beverages.

Iodine

Iodine is essential for the production of thyroid hormones, which in turn are essential for growth and development, protein synthesis, and other important bodily functions.

Deficiency of this trace mineral results in goiter, a condition that causes enlargement of the thyroid gland. Overconsumption can also cause thyroid gland enlargement.

Dietary Sources Include: Seafood, iodized salt, egg yolks, and iodine-fortified foods and beverages. Iodine can also enter the diet through a variety of other food-related avenues, including the use of iodine-containing additives in feed for cattle and chickens and the use of iodine-containing

---

[90] Aiken, Janet S. Nutritional Science: Concepts, Controversies, and Therapies. p. 197. Copyright © 2008 Janet S. Aiken, Ph.D., Date Palm Press, Boca Raton, Florida.
[91] Grosvenor, Mary B. and Smolin, Lori A. Nutrition From Science To Life. p. 454. ©2002 Harcourt, Inc. Reproduced with permission of John Wiley and Sons, Inc.
[92] Bleys, J., et al., "Selenium and Diabetes: More Bad News for Supplements," *Annals of Internal Medicine,"* August 21, 2007, Volume 147, Issue 4.

disinfectants on cows and in milking machines and storage tanks; the use of iodine-containing sterilizing agents in fast-food restaurants; and the addition of iodine to dough conditioners and some food colorings.[93]

Fluoride

Fluoride helps prevent dental caries (cavities). Its use as an additive in toothpaste, mouthwash, water, and pesticides, however, is controversial, as it is not an essential nutrient and can be toxic. While fluoride deficiency may lead to tooth or bone problems, consuming high doses of fluoride can have the same or similar effects and can also cause other serious adverse effects.

Cooking in aluminum may reduce the fluoride content of foods.[94] Consuming fluoride-rich foods or beverages together with calcium-rich foods (such as when tea is consumed with milk or cream), decreases fluoride absorption in the body.

Dietary Sources Include: Fluoride is found in small amounts in most foods and in greater amounts in fluoride toothpastes, fluoridated water, foods prepared with fluoridated water, some teas, and fish with bones. Foods cooked in Teflon® may also pick up fluoride.[95]

Chromium

Chromium is essential for the normal utilization of glucose. It is also needed for the metabolism of both fats and protein. The form of chromium

---

[93] Grosvenor, Mary B. and Smolin, Lori A. <u>Nutrition From Science To Life</u>. p. 455.
©2002 Harcourt, Inc. Reproduced with permission of John Wiley and Sons, Inc.
[94] Full, C.A. and Parkins, Frederick M., "Effect of Cooking Vessel Composition on Fluoride," *Journal of Dental Research,* 54:192. Copyright © 1975 International & American Associations for Dental Research. Reprinted by Permission of SAGE Publications.
[95] See footnote 94.

found in foods and used by the body is called trivalent chromium, written as "chromium (III)."

Chromium deficiency is uncommon in this country, though those who are malnourished or are taking medications that interfere with chromium absorption are at risk. Taking excessive amounts of chromium can be toxic. The chromium picolinate form of chromium has been shown to damage DNA in laboratory-grown cells.[96]

Dietary Sources Include: Whole grains, nuts, liver, brewer's yeast, and chromium-fortified foods and beverages. The use of stainless steel cookware and utensils can also add chromium to the diet, as it leaches from the steel into foods during cooking.

Molybdenum

Like zinc and several other minerals, molybdenum is essential in the activation of certain bodily enzymes. It is also needed for the synthesis and activity of various other compounds in the body including those that are components of our DNA and RNA.

Molybdenum deficiency is rare, though those who are malnourished may be at risk. The risk of toxicity appears to be low. The Food and Nutrition Board of the Institute of Medicine has set a UL for molybdenum use in adults 19 years and older at 2 mg daily.[97]

Dietary Sources Include: Lentils, beans, peas, whole grains, nuts, milk, cheese, liver, and molybdenum-fortified foods and beverages.

[96] Grosvenor, Mary B. and Smolin, Lori A. Nutrition From Science To Life. p. 501. ©2002 Harcourt, Inc. Reproduced with permission of John Wiley and Sons, Inc.
[97] "Molybdenum," Dietary Reference Intakes for Vitamin A, Vitamin K, Arsenic, Boron, Chromium, Copper, Iodine, Iron, Manganese, Molybdenum, Nickel, Silicon, Vanadium, and Zinc, p. 420. Reprinted with permission from the National Academies Press. Copyright © 2000 National Academy of Sciences.

Other Trace Elements
A variety of other elements are found in small amounts in the body. Many of them are being researched for their potential beneficial roles in human health when consumed at very low levels. Those that have been reviewed include arsenic, boron, nickel, silicon, and vanadium.[98] Aluminum, bromine, cadmium, germanium, lead, lithium, rubidium, and tin—most of which are known to be toxic at higher levels—may also play important roles in the body when consumed in extremely minute quantities, though sufficient research has yet to be done in these areas.

Toxic Minerals
The heavy metals lead, mercury, cadmium, inorganic arsenic, and aluminum are toxic even when consumed at relatively low levels and can displace or replace beneficial minerals in the body. Organic forms of arsenic, which occur naturally in dairy products, oils, meat, fish, shellfish, and other foods are an exception, as they are considered to be much less toxic than inorganic forms of arsenic (such as those used for industrial wood applications).

For more detailed information on minerals in general visit **http://lpi.oregonstate.edu/infocenter/minerals.html**.

To see the values for 19 nutrients in over 1,274 foods visit:
http://www.nal.usda.gov/fnic/foodcomp/Data/HG72/hg72_2002.pdf

Enzymes
Enzymes have a variety of functions in the body, including facilitating digestion and acting as antioxidants. Digestive enzymes, for example, break

---

[98] See footnote 97.

down sugars, fats, proteins, and related compounds for use as energy. There are over a dozen different digestive enzymes found naturally in our digestive secretions. These enzymes can also be obtained as supplements, either individually or in combination with other enzymes.

Some enzymes are also found in foods, such as papain in papaya and bromelain in pineapple. Enzymes found in foods are only active when a food is raw, however, as they are destroyed by cooking.

Enzymes that break down proteins include pepsin, trypsin, chymotripsin, and rennin. Enzymes that break down sugars include amylase, sucrase, lactase, maltase, and dextromase. The main enzyme involved in the breakdown of fats is lipase.

Other enzymes, namely superoxide dismutase (SOD), glutathione peroxidase, and catalase, act as antioxidants.

Phytochemicals (Phytonutrients)

Phytochemicals, also called phytonutrients, are plant-based food substances that have either been proven to have health benefits or are believed to have them. Phytosterols, for example, are plant sterols with a chemical structure similar to that of cholesterol. They are believed to help lower blood cholesterol levels by inhibiting the absorption of intestinal cholesterol.[99] They are found in a variety of snack foods, beverages, margarines, and spreads.

Other phytochemicals include carotenoids, flavonoids, phytoestrogens, saponins, glucosinolates, sulfides, and tannins.

Zoochemicals

Zoochemicals are animal-based food substances, that, like phytonutrients, have either been proven to have or are believed to have health-promoting qualities. They include the omega-3 fatty acids EPA (eicosapentaenoic acid)

---

[99] Ostlund, Richard E., "Phytosterols in Human Nutrition." Reprinted with permission from the *Annual Review of Nutrition,* Volume 22, ©2002 by Annual Reviews. www.annualreviews.org.

and DHA (docosahexaenoic acid) which are found in fatty fish such as sardines, mackerel, salmon, and tuna.

Amino acids

Amino acids are the chemical building blocks that make up proteins. As supplements, they are often promoted to athletes as a way to build endurance, enhance muscle growth, and lessen fatigue, among other things. However, the overall use of amino acids is not recommended for the following three reasons: 1) there is little verified scientific evidence that amino acids benefit athletes; 2) the consumption of high doses of amino acids may interfere with the absorption of other amino acids and nutrients in the diet; and 3) there have been several reports of illness due to contaminants found in amino acid supplements.[100]

Amino acids are also used medicinally for treating a variety of health problems. The supplementation of essential amino acids may be required during illness.

Antioxidants

Antioxidants protect the body from cellular damage caused by dietary and environmental hazards such as rancid fats and cigarette smoke. They exist in the form of vitamins, vitamin precursors, minerals, enzymes, and phytochemicals. Vitamins C and E and beta-carotene (a vitamin A precursor) are prime examples. Although taking antioxidants in supplement form may provide health benefits, consuming foods that contain antioxidants often offers compound benefits.

Essential fatty acids (EFAs)

Fatty acids make up fats. They are involved in growth and development, including that of the eyes, skin, and brain, and are important to good heart health.

---

[100] Grosvenor, Mary B. and Smolin, Lori A. Nutrition From Science To Life. p. 504. ©2002 Harcourt, Inc. Reproduced with permission of John Wiley and Sons, Inc.

The body is capable of manufacturing most of the fatty acids it needs to run efficiently. Only two — alpha-linolenic acid (an omega-3 fatty acid) and linoleic acid (an omega-6 fatty acid) — must be obtained from foods or supplements. Because the body cannot manufacture either of these fatty acids, they are referred to as essential fatty acids, or EFAs.

The consumption of alpha-linolenic acid and linoleic acid supports the production of other important omega-3 and omega-6 fatty acids. Alpha-linolenic acid produces EPA and DHA; linoleic acid produces arachidonic acid. When the level of either alpha-linolenic or linoleic acid in the body is inadequate, the other fatty acids they support also become essential.

In addition to supplements, good sources of omega-3 fatty acids include salmon and other fatty fish; flaxseed (linseed); and canola, flaxseed, and soybean oils. Good sources of omega-6 fatty acids include oils from wheat germ, soybeans, corn, sunflowers, safflowers, and evening primrose.

Herbs

Herbs have been used medicinally for centuries. Today there are not only thousands of herbs to choose from, but also an extensive selection of herbal supplements and dietary aids. **It is important that they be used with caution.** Potency, origin, and authenticity are only a few related concerns, as are medication interactions and the age and sex of the consumer. There are also considerations regarding the use of pesticides, herbicides, and other chemicals used for herb growth.

Many herbs are replacements for drugs. Some are stronger than drugs, or can enhance drugs, causing unwanted, unexpected, or even dangerous effects. For example, St. John's Wort should not be taken before surgery as it can prolong and intensify the effects of both narcotics and anesthesia. The effects of all herbs should be carefully researched prior to use.

To view fact sheets that provide information on commonly used herbs visit
the National Institutes of Health at
http://nccam.nih.gov/health/herbsataglance.htm

Glyconutrients

Glyconutrients are relatively new to the nutrient scene. They are a group of eight simple sugars (monosaccharides) which may help the body form glycoproteins (protein molecules with sugar molecules attached). Glycoproteins help cells communicate with each other and can therefore enhance health. The body produces glycoproteins on its own from various foods, therefore supplemental glyconutrients may be unnecessary when a balanced diet is being consumed.

Probiotics

The large intestine is host to hundreds of species of beneficial bacteria. These microorganisms, known collectively as intestinal microflora, can be affected by diet, stress, antibiotics, and our overall state of health.

Probiotics are beneficial bacteria that help to maintain or restore our intestinal microflora. They include lactobacillus and bifidobacterium, among others, and are found in yogurt and other foods (especially fermented dairy foods) as well as in a variety of supplemental forms.

Studies have shown numerous potential benefits from the use of probiotics, including lowered cholesterol; enhanced immunity; treatment of diarrhea and irritable bowel syndrome; a reduction in the recurrence of bladder cancer; and the prevention and management of eczema in children. [101,102]

Prebiotics

Prebiotics are substances that provide an effective food source for beneficial bacteria already present in the colon. An example is fructooligosaccharides (FOS). Onions, garlic, asparagus, artichokes, and bananas are natural sources of FOS, while commercially produced FOS is added to a variety of products from children's chewable vitamins to powdered drink mixes.

---

[101] St.-Onge, M.P., et al., "Consumption of fermented and nonfermented dairy products effects on cholesterol concentrations and metabolism," *American Journal of Clinical Nutrition,* 2000; 71:674-681.
[102] National Institutes of Health, "An Introduction to Probiotics," *NCCAM Publication No.* D345, August 2008, <http://nccam.nih.gov/health/probiotics> (December 13, 2008).

Protein

Protein is often supplemented in the diet through the use of powders, beverages, and nutrition bars. While in some cases this is done in place of eating prepared meals, in many others it is done in an effort to build additional muscle. However, once the body's protein needs have been met, adding more protein will not add more muscle. It can, however, lead to weight gain if it is consumed on a regular basis, and may also promote dehydration.[103]

Other Nutritional Supplements

There are numerous other types of nutritional supplements. Some have been proven to be beneficial or potentially beneficial, while many others have not. For example, bee pollen and royal jelly are sold as supplements even though there is a lack of scientific evidence that they provide any tangible health benefits (for more information on this topic visit **http://edis. ifas.ufl.edu/AA158)**. Further, their strong potential to cause allergic reactions is a serious concern. With all nutritional supplements it is important to thoroughly check on both their potential and proven effects before use.

---

[103] Grosvenor, Mary B. and Smolin, Lori A. <u>Nutrition From Science To Life</u>. p. 197. © 2002 Harcourt, Inc. Reproduced with permission of John Wiley and Sons, Inc.

Chapter 9

The Centers for Disease Control and Prevention estimate that 76 million people get sick, 325,000 are hospitalized, and 5,000 die each year in the U.S. from foodborne illness. These statistics all too vividly emphasize the importance of food safety. At every stage of the food chain—from production, shipping, and storage to preparation and consumption—effective methods of inspection, handling, and sanitation are critical to ensure protection against pathogens and toxins and reduce related health risks. Knowledge about food safety and attention to detail are equally essential. These factors are important regardless of whether we are a farmer, butcher, chef, or consumer—or anyone in between who handles or consumes food.

Technology also plays a major role in food safety, as well as in enhancing the nutritional value and availability of foods. The goals of nutritional technology are to provide the safest, freshest, most nutritious foods and related products in sufficient quantities to feed the growing population. These goals are achieved via a working combination of human effort, food safety programs, machinery, and science. Technology doesn't always come without risks, however. Here we look at food safety and technology, how they are related, and potential problems and benefits we may encounter in these areas in the future.

Food Safety

The U.S. food supply is one of the safest in the world. Despite this fact, the increasing number of laboratory-confirmed cases of foodborne illness over the past few years—particularly those caused by E. coli[1] and Vibrio[2]—has

[1] Centers for Disease Control and Prevention, "FoodNet Facts and Figures - Incidence trends, 2007," March 2008, <http://www.cdc.gov/foodnet/factsandfigures/10.pdf> (December 12, 2008).
[2] Centers for Disease Control and Prevention, *MMWR Weekly,* April 13, 2007, 56(14); 336-339, <http://www.cdc.gov/mmwr/preview/mmwrhtml/mm5614a4.htm> (December 12, 2008>.

caused growing concern among consumers and regulators alike. The causes are varied and include changes in food production and packaging; food handling errors; increased consumption of imported foods; increased consumption of raw meats and seafood; and a rise in the population of both elderly and immunocompromised individuals. The situation has caused consumers to be more alert to food safety and recalls, and has prompted regulators to rethink and restructure the way they monitor foods and control outbreaks.

Much remains to be done to reach the overall national health objectives for foodborne illnesses. Enhanced measures are needed to control pathogens in plants and animals; reduce or prevent contamination during growing, harvesting, and processing; and educate consumers more effectively about risks and preventive measures. Such measures can be better focused when the source of human infections (e.g., plant or animal species and transmission route) is known. In particular, further research is needed to understand how contamination of fresh produce occurs so that new measures to reduce such contamination can be developed and effectively implemented.

Food Safety Regulation in the U.S.: An Overview
The FDA, USDA, EPA, and NOAA work individually and collaboratively to ensure food safety from a variety of angles (for details on their individual and joint roles, as well as contact information, see chapter three). Within this system, the FDA carries responsibility for the bulk of regulatory enforcement. Under federal law, the agency is required to protect public health by ensuring safe handling—including production, processing, packaging, shipment, and storage—of all domestic and imported foods other than those solely under the jurisdiction of the USDA. It is also responsible for overseeing the safety of ingredients (including additives) used in food products, as well as the safety of infant formulas, medical foods, and dietary supplements. However, as the FDA's policing capabilities are limited, even the agency's most well-intentioned goals have the potential to go unmet. In effect, most food and beverage manufacturers, as well as those who produce nutritional supplements, are on their honor when it comes to proper

production and accurate labeling (for more on labeling see chapter twelve). Funding is a major issue, affecting the number of qualified professionals on staff at the FDA, the amount of nutritional education the agency disperses to the public, and the amount of food-related research it initiates. This is evident in the fact that while consumers are usually made aware of food and drug interactions and interactions between over-the-counter and prescription drugs, there are currently more than 3000 food additives[3] in use on the market and not one of them has been sufficiently tested and publicly reported on for possible effects when combined with other additives. To further complicate the situation, new foods, drugs, and food additives continue to flood the market, creating an immense backlog.

Common Causes of Foodborne Illness

A number of different pathogens, including bacteria, toxins, viruses, fungi, and parasites, can cause foodborne illness. Listed here are some of the more common of these pathogens, how they are known or believed to be transmitted, and ways to avoid them.

Bacteria

Campylobacter
Campylobacter jejuni is a bacterial pathogen that causes fever, diarrhea, and abdominal cramps and may be a precipitating factor in Guillain-Barre syndrome. According to the CDC, it is the most commonly identified bacterial cause of diarrheal illness in the world. These bacteria live in the intestines of healthy birds, and most raw poultry meat has C. jejuni on it. Eating raw or undercooked chicken, or other food that has been contaminated with juices dripping from raw chicken, is the most frequent source of this infection. Careful handling and thorough cooking of chicken and poultry products along with

---

[3] U.S. Food and Drug Administration, "EAFUS: A Food Additive Database," October 17, 2008, <http://www.cfsan.fda.gov/~dms/eafus.html> (December 12, 2008).

proper disinfection of all surfaces they come in contact with are effective ways to avoid this common foodborne pathogen.

Salmonella

Like Campylobacter, salmonella is a bacterium that is widespread in the intestines of birds. It is also widespread in the intestines of reptiles and mammals. It can spread to humans via a variety of different foods of animal origin, including eggs, meat, poultry, and unpasteurized dairy products such as raw milk and cheese. It can also be found in fish, shrimp, frog legs, yeast, coconut, sauces, sprouts, salad dressing, cake mixes, cream-filled desserts, toppings, dried gelatin, peanut butter, cocoa, and chocolate. The illness it causes, salmonellosis, typically includes fever, diarrhea, and abdominal cramps. In those who are immunocompromised it can invade the bloodstream and cause life-threatening infections. Thorough cooking of foods effectively kills salmonella bacteria.

Escherichia coli 0157:H7

Escherichia coli O157:H7 is a bacterial pathogen associated with cattle and other similar animals. It is just one of several forms of E. coli. Human illness typically follows consumption of food or water that has been contaminated with microscopic amounts of cow feces. Raw hamburger (ground beef) has been the source of many documented outbreaks, though alfalfa sprouts, lettuce, raw milk, unpasteurized fruit juices, dry-cured salami, and game meats have also been implicated. Characteristic symptoms include severe bloody diarrhea and painful abdominal cramps which may be accompanied by fever. In approximately 3% to 5% of cases, a serious complication known as hemolytic uremic syndrome (HUS) occurs several weeks after the initial onset of symptoms. HUS causes temporary anemia, profuse bleeding, and kidney failure. It is more common among children than adults. Careful handling and thorough cooking of ground meats, thorough washing and drying (with paper towels) of produce, and avoidance of unpasteurized dairy products and fruit juices can help reduce the incidence of E. coli.

Vibrio

Vibrio vulnificus is a bacterium in the same family as those that cause cholera. It normally lives in warm seawater and is part of a group of vibrios that are called "halophilic" because they require salt to exist. V. vulnificus can cause disease in those who eat contaminated seafood, particularly oysters, though it can also be transmitted via an open wound that is exposed to seawater. Among healthy people, ingestion of V. vulnificus can cause vomiting, diarrhea, and abdominal pain within 16 hours. In immunocompromised persons, particularly those with chronic liver disease, V. vulnificus can infect the bloodstream, causing a severe and life-threatening illness characterized by fever, chills, decreased blood pressure (septic shock), and blistering skin lesions. V. vulnificus bloodstream infections are fatal about 50% of the time. Vibrio does not affect the appearance, taste, or odor of oysters. The CDC recommends the following ways to lessen the risk of contracting a V. vulnificus infection:

- Avoid eating raw oysters or other raw shellfish.
- Cook shellfish (oysters, clams, mussels) thoroughly.
- For shellfish in the shell, either a) boil until the shells open and continue boiling for 5 more minutes, or b) steam until the shells open and then continue cooking for 9 more minutes.
- **Do not eat those shellfish that do not open during cooking.** Boil shucked oysters at least 3 minutes, or fry them in oil at least 10 minutes at 375 °F.
- Avoid cross-contamination of cooked seafood and other foods with raw seafood and juices from raw seafood.
- Eat shellfish promptly after cooking and refrigerate leftovers.
- Avoid exposure of open wounds or broken skin to warm salt water or brackish water, or to raw shellfish harvested from such waters.
- Wear protective clothing (e.g., gloves) when handling raw shellfish.

Shigella

Shigella are a group of bacteria that cause the infectious disease shigellosis. Shigellosis can be acquired from eating contaminated food (which usually looks and smells normal) or drinking contaminated water. Vegetables can become contaminated with Shigella if they are harvested from a field with sewage in it, flies can breed in Shigella-infected feces and then contaminate food, and water may become contaminated if sewage runs into it. Food may also become contaminated by infected food handlers who forget to wash their hands thoroughly with soap after using the bathroom.

Most who are infected with Shigella develop diarrhea, fever, and stomach cramps starting a day or two after exposure to the bacteria. The diarrhea is often bloody. Shigellosis usually resolves in 5 to 7 days. Persons with shigellosis in the U.S. rarely require hospitalization. A severe infection with high fever may be accompanied by seizures in children less than 2 years old. Some persons who are infected may have no symptoms at all, but may still pass the Shigella bacteria to others. Frequent and thorough hand washing with soap (especially during food handling and preparation) and thorough washing and drying of produce (with paper towels) can help reduce the incidence of shigellosis.

Listeria

Listeria monocytogenes is a hardy bacterium found in soil and water that can readily transfer to plants, animals, birds, and humans. Unlike most other pathogenic bacteria that multiply at room temperature (most double in number every 30 to 40 minutes), it can grow in temperatures as low as 3 °C (37.4 °F), making refrigerators and freezers excellent breeding grounds. It has been found in a variety of raw foods, such as uncooked meats and vegetables, as well as in processed foods that become contaminated after processing, such as soft cheeses, cold cuts, and hot dogs. Unpasteurized (raw) milk or foods made from unpasteurized milk can also contain the bacterium, as can vegetables that have been exposed to contaminated soil or manure used as fertilizer. Animals can carry the bacterium without appearing ill and can contaminate meats, dairy products, and other foods of pearing ill and can contaminate meats, dairy products, and other foods of animal origin.

According to the CDC, listeriosis, a serious infection caused by eating food contaminated with L. monocytogenes, has recently been recognized as an important public health problem in the United States. The disease primarily affects the elderly, pregnant women (who are about 20 times more likely to contract listeriosis than other healthy adults), newborns, and adults with weakened immune systems (who are about 300 times more likely to contract listeriosis than those with normal immune systems). Although rare, persons without these risk factors can also be affected.

Listeriosis can cause septicemia (blood poisoning), meningitis (or meningoencephalitis), encephalitis, and intrauterine or cervical infections in pregnant women, which may result in spontaneous abortion (2nd/3rd trimester) or stillbirth. The onset of these disorders is usually preceded by flu-like symptoms including persistent fever. Gastrointestinal symptoms such as nausea, vomiting, and diarrhea may precede more serious forms of listeriosis or may be the only symptoms experienced. The onset time to serious forms of listeriosis is unknown but may range from a few days to three weeks. The onset time to gastrointestinal symptoms is also unknown but is probably greater than 12 hours.

Listeria is killed by pasteurization and cooking; however, in certain ready-to-eat foods such as hot dogs and deli meats contamination may occur after cooking but before packaging. The risk of contracting listeriosis can be reduced by avoidance of high-risk foods, frequent hand washing with soap, thorough cooking of foods, and careful food handling. The CDC offers the following specific recommendations:

General recommendations

- Thoroughly cook raw food from animal sources, such as beef, pork, or poultry.
- Wash raw vegetables thoroughly before eating.
- Keep uncooked meats separate from vegetables, cooked foods, and ready-to-eat foods.

- Avoid unpasteurized (raw) milk or foods made from unpasteurized milk.
- Wash hands, cutting boards, and all utensils after handling uncooked foods.
- Consume perishable and ready-to-eat foods as soon as possible.

Recommendations (in addition to those listed above) for persons at high risk, such as pregnant women and those with weakened immune systems:

- Do not eat hot dogs, luncheon meats, or deli meats, unless they are re-heated until steaming hot.
- Avoid getting fluid from hot dog packages on other foods, utensils, and food preparation surfaces, and wash hands after handling hot dogs, luncheon meats, and deli meats.
- Do not eat soft cheeses such as feta, Brie, and Camembert, blue-veined cheeses, or Mexican-style cheeses such as queso blanco, queso fresco, and Panela, unless they have labels that clearly state they are made from pasteurized milk.
- Do not eat refrigerated pâtés or meat spreads. Canned or shelf-stable pâtés and meat spreads may be an option.
- Do not eat refrigerated smoked seafood, unless it is contained in a cooked dish, such as a casserole. This includes salmon, trout, whitefish, cod, tuna, or mackerel that is labeled "nova-style," "lox," "kippered," "smoked," or "jerky." Canned or shelf-stable smoked seafood may be an option.

Yersinia

Yersinia enterocolitica is one of three pathogenic bacterium of the genus Yersinia. It can be found in contaminated meat (especially raw or under-cooked pork, including chitterlings), oysters, fish, and raw milk, as well as in contaminated water. It is the cause of the infectious disease yersiniosis. Infection with Y. enterocolitica can cause a variety of symptoms depending on the age of the person infected. Infection occurs most often in young children. Common symptoms in children are fever, abdominal pain, and diarrhea, which is often bloody. Symptoms typically develop 4 to 7 days after exposure and may last 1 to 3 weeks or longer. In older children and adults, right-side abdominal pain and fever may be the predominant symptoms, and may be confused with appendicitis. In a small proportion of cases, complications such as skin rash, joint pains, or spread of bacteria to the bloodstream can occur. The CDC suggests doing the following to avoid exposure:

• Avoid eating raw or undercooked pork.

• Consume only pasteurized milk or milk products.

• Wash hands with soap and water before eating and preparing food, after contact with animals, and after handling raw meat.

• After handling raw pork chitterlings, clean hands and fingernails scrupulously with soap and water. This is especially important before touching infants or their toys, bottles, or pacifiers.

• Prevent cross-contamination in the kitchen: Use separate cutting boards for meat and other foods and carefully clean all cutting boards, countertops, and utensils with soap and hot water after preparing raw meat.

• Dispose of animal feces in a sanitary manner.

Staphylococcus aureus

Staphylococcus aureus is a bacterium of which seven strains are capable of producing a highly heat-stable protein toxin that causes staphylococcal food poisoning (staphyloenterotoxicosis, staphyloenterotoxemia) in humans. These toxins are both salt tolerant and heat resistant and cannot be destroyed by cooking. Food poisoning caused by this bacterium is not contagious. Foods that frequently cause staphylococcal food poisoning include meat and meat products; poultry and egg products; salads such as egg, tuna, chicken, potato, and macaroni; bakery products such as cream-filled pastries, cream pies, and chocolate eclairs; sandwich fillings; and milk and dairy products, including cheese. Foods that require considerable handling during preparation and that are kept at slightly elevated temperatures after preparation are frequently involved in staphylococcal food poisoning.

The onset of symptoms in staphylococcal food poisoning is usually rapid and in many cases intense, depending on individual susceptibility to the toxin, the amount of contaminated food eaten, the amount of toxin in the food ingested, and the general health of the victim. The most common symptoms are nausea, vomiting, retching, abdominal cramping, and exhaustion. Some individuals may not demonstrate all the symptoms associated with the illness. In more severe cases, headache, muscle cramping, and transient changes in blood pressure and pulse rate may occur. Recovery generally takes two days; however, it is not unusual for complete recovery to take three days and sometimes longer in severe cases.

In order to avoid this type of food poisoning, it is important to prevent the contamination of food with S. aureus before the toxin can be produced. The CDC makes the following recommendations to reduce incidence and exposure:

- Wash hands and under fingernails vigorously with soap and water before handling and preparing food.
- Do not prepare food if you have a nose or eye infection.
- Do not prepare or serve food for others if you have wounds or skin infections on your hands or wrists.
- Keep kitchens and food-serving areas clean and sanitized.
- If food is to be stored longer than two hours, keep hot foods hot (over 140 °F) and cold foods cold (40 °F or under).
- Store cooked food in a wide, shallow container and refrigerate as soon as possible.

Parasites

Giardia
Giardia intestinalis (also known as Giardia lamblia) is a one-celled microscopic parasite that causes giardiasis, a diarrheal illness. It is found in contaminated foods and water. Once an animal or person has been infected with G. intestinalis, the parasite lives in the intestine and is passed in the

stool. Because the parasite is protected by an outer shell, it can survive outside the body and in the environment for long periods of time. During the past 2 decades, Giardia infection has become recognized as one of the most common causes of waterborne disease (found in both drinking water and recreational water) in humans in the United States. Giardia are found worldwide and within every region of the United States.

The onset of illness is usually within one week of exposure and may involve diarrhea. The illness normally lasts for 1 to 2 weeks, but there are cases of chronic infections lasting months to years.

The best ways to avoid exposure to G. intestinalis are to thoroughly wash hands with soap on a regular basis and stay alert to any community-wide outbreaks of disease related to drinking or recreational water.

Viruses

Noroviruses

Also called caliciviruses, this viral group that includes the Norwalk virus and Norwalk-like viruses is an extremely common cause of foodborne illness. These viruses are rarely diagnosed, however, because the laboratory test to detect them is not widely available. Each virus causes an acute gastrointestinal illness that can include nausea, vomiting, diarrhea, and stomach cramping, and is often referred to as the "stomach flu." This generally resolves within two days, though it is highly contagious from the onset of symptoms to as long as two weeks after recovery. Unlike many foodborne pathogens that spread via animals, it is believed that Norwalk-like viruses spread primarily from one infected person to another. Infected kitchen workers can contaminate a salad or sandwich as they prepare it if they have the virus on their hands. Infected fishermen have contaminated oysters as they harvested them. These recommendations can help reduce the incidence of noroviruses:

- Frequently wash your hands, especially after bathroom visits and changing diapers and before eating or preparing food.

213

- Carefully wash fruits and vegetables, and steam oysters before eating them.
- Thoroughly clean and disinfect contaminated surfaces immediately after an episode of illness by using a bleach-based household cleaner.

Hepatitis A Virus

Hepatitis A Virus is excreted in the feces of infected people and can produce clinical disease when susceptible individuals consume contaminated water or foods. It is characterized by sudden onset of fever, malaise, nausea, anorexia, and abdominal discomfort, followed in several days by jaundice. Cold cuts and sandwiches, fruits and fruit juices, milk and milk products, vegetables, salads, shellfish, and iced drinks are commonly implicated in outbreaks. Water, shellfish, and salads are the most frequent sources. Contamination of foods by infected workers in food processing plants and restaurants is common. Proper hygiene, including thorough hand washing with soap, is essential to reduce the incidence of exposure.

Natural Toxins

Ciguatera

Ciguatera fish poisoning, also referred to simply as ciguatera, is an illness caused by eating subtropical and tropical marine fish that contain toxins produced by a microalgae called Gambierdiscus toxicus. The most common fish to carry ciguatoxins are groupers, barracudas, snappers, jacks, hogfish, mackerel, sea bass, mullet, and triggerfish, though many other species of warm-water fishes harbor them. The occurrence of toxic fish is sporadic, and not all fish of a given species or from a given locality will be toxic.

Those who have ciguatera may experience nausea, vomiting, and neurologic symptoms such as numbness or tingling (parasthesia) of the lips, fingers, or toes within six hours of consumption of toxic fish. They also may experience temperature reversal, in which cold things feel hot and hot things feel cold, as well as a variety of other symptoms including dizziness, muscle weakness, low blood pressure, and cardiovascular disturbances. There is no cure for ciguatera. Symptoms usually go away in days or weeks but have lasted for years in some individuals. In a few isolated cases neurological symptoms have persisted for several years, and in other cases recovered patients have experienced recurrence of neurological symptoms months to years after recovery. Such relapses are most often associated with changes in dietary habits or with consumption of alcohol. Ciguatera is related with a low incidence of death resulting from respiratory and cardiovascular failure. Consuming fish from known safe sources, staying alert to ciguatoxin advisories for certain fishing areas, and avoiding consumption of whole fish (particularly internal organs) and large reef fish may help to lessen the risk of contracting ciguatera. Visit **http://www.rsmas.miami.edu/ groups/niehs/science/ciguatera.htm** for more information about this toxin.

Shellfish Toxins

There are four types of shellfish poisoning:

- Paralytic Shellfish Poisoning (PSP)
- Diarrhetic Shellfish Poisoning (DSP)
- Neurotoxic Shellfish Poisoning (NSP)
- Amnesic Shellfish Poisoning (ASP)

Paralytic shellfish poisoning is caused by 20 different algal toxins that are derivatives of saxitoxin. The algae associated with these toxins have a red-brown color and can grow to such numbers that they cause red streaks to appear in the ocean called "red tides." This toxin is known to concentrate within certain shellfish that typically live in the colder coastal waters of the Pacific states and New England, though the syndrome has been reported in Central America as well. Shellfish that have caused this disease include mussels, cockles, clams, scallops, oysters, crabs, and lobsters. Symptoms begin anywhere from 15 minutes to 10 hours after eating the contaminated shellfish, although they usually occur within 2 hours. Symptoms are generally mild, and begin with numbness or tingling of the face, arms, and legs. This is followed by headache, dizziness, nausea, and muscular incoordination.

Patients sometimes describe a floating sensation. In cases of severe poisoning, muscle paralysis and respiratory failure occur, and in these cases death may occur in 2 to 25 hours.

Diarrhetic shellfish poisoning is not common to the U.S., but rather has been experienced in Europe. Not only does this type of poisoning cause diarrhea, but the toxins associated with it have been reported to be tumor-promoting agents.[4] Affected shellfish include mussels, oysters, and scallops.

Neurotoxic shellfish poisoning is caused by yet another type of algae with a toxin that occasionally accumulates in oysters, clams, and mussels from the Gulf of Mexico and the Atlantic coast of the southern states, including Florida. Symptoms begin 1 to 3 hours after eating the contaminated shellfish and include numbness, tingling in the mouth, arms and legs, incoordination, and gastrointestinal upset. As in ciguatera poisoning, some patients report temperature reversal. Death is rare. Recovery normally occurs in 2 to 3 days.

Amnesic shellfish poisoning is a rare syndrome caused by a toxin made by a microscopic red-brown saltwater plant, or diatom, called Nitzchia pungens. The toxin produced by these diatoms is concentrated in shellfish such as mussels. Patients first experience gastrointestinal distress within 24 hours after eating contaminated shellfish. Other reported symptoms have included dizziness, headache, disorientation, and permanent short-term memory loss. In severe cases of poisoning, seizures, focal weakness (or paralysis), and death may occur.

Avoiding the consumption of shellfish from restricted areas, such as those with red tide, can reduce the risk of shellfish poisoning. For more information on the incidence of red tide visit **http://www.whoi.edu/ oceanus/viewArticle.do?id=47406**.

---

[4] National Oceanic and Atmospheric Administration, NWSC, "Harmful Algal Blooms," n.d., <http:// www. nwfsc.noaa.gov/hab/habs_toxins/marine_biotoxins/dsp/index.html> (December 12, 2008).

Scombroid Poisoning

Scombrotoxic fish poisoning also known as scombroid or histamine fish poisoning, is caused by bacterial spoilage of certain finfish such as tuna, mackerel, bonito, mahi-mahi, sardines, amberjack, and, rarely, other fish. As bacteria break down fish proteins, byproducts such as histamine and other substances that block histamine breakdown build up in fish. Eating spoiled fish that have high levels of these histamines can cause human disease. Symptoms begin within 2 minutes to 2 hours after eating spoiled fish. The most common symptoms are rash, diarrhea, flushing, sweating, headache, and vomiting. Burning or swelling of the mouth, abdominal pain, or a metallic taste may also occur. The majority of patients have mild symptoms that resolve within a few hours. Treatment is generally unnecessary, but antihistamines or epinephrine may be needed in certain instances. Symptoms may be more severe in patients taking certain medications that slow the breakdown of histamine by their liver, such as isoniazide and doxycycline. **Cooking does not remove the toxin.** According to the CDC the only effective method for prevention of scombroid fish poisoning is consistent temperature control of fish at ≤ 40 °F (≤ 4.4 °C) at all times between catching and consumption. Safe consumption of fish in general can be promoted by following these points regarding freshness:

- Fish must be **refrigerated or properly iced**. When iced, it should be displayed on a thick bed of fresh ice that is not melting, preferably in a case or under some type of cover.
- Fish should **smell fresh and mild,** not fishy, sour, or ammonia-like.
- A fish's **eyes should be clear** and bulge a little (except for a few naturally cloudy-eyed fish, such as walleye pike).
- Whole fish and filets should have **firm, shiny flesh** and bright red gills free from slime. Dull flesh could mean the fish is old. Note: Fish fillets that have been previously frozen may have lost some of their shine, but they are fine to eat.
- The flesh should spring back when pressed.

- Fish fillets should display **no darkening or drying** around the edges. They should have no green or yellowish discoloration, and should not appear dry or mushy in any areas.

Chemical Toxins

There are many chemical toxins used on foods, most of which are for purposes of pest control. In some cases foods have both natural and chemical toxins. Potatoes, for example, are often treated with sprout inhibitors to stop the development of dangerous natural toxins such as solanine. This must be carefully regulated, however. In one case, a Cornell University biochemist found residues from sprout inhibitors on potato peels four times greater than what government guidelines allow for whole potatoes.[5]

Other Pathogens

Prions
Prions are normal proteins of animal tissues that can misfold and become infectious. They are not cellular organisms, nor are they viruses. Prions are associated with a group of diseases called Transmissible Spongiform Encephalopathies (TSEs). In humans, the illness suspected of being foodborne is variant Creutzfeldt-Jakob disease (vCJD). The human disease vCJD and the cattle disease, bovine spongiform encephalopathy (BSE), also known as "mad cow" disease, appear to be caused by the same agent. Other similar but not identical TSE diseases exist in animals, but there is no known transmission of these TSEs to humans.

The major concern for consumers is the potential contamination of meat products by BSE-contaminated tissues or the inclusion of BSE-contaminated tissues in foods or dietary supplements. High risk tissues for BSE contamination include the cattle's skull, brain, trigeminal ganglia (nerves attached to the brain, eyes, tonsils, spinal cord), dorsal root ganglia (nerves attached to the spinal cord), and the distal ileum (part of the small intestine).

---

[5] "Peel your potatoes to avoid toxins, says Cornell Researcher," *Environmental Nutrition,* February 1993.

The direct or indirect intake of high-risk tissues may have been the source of human illnesses in the United Kingdom and elsewhere. Bovine meat (if free of central nervous system tissue) and milk have, to date, shown no infectivity in test animals. Gelatin, derived from the hides and bones of cattle, appears to be very low risk, especially when adequate attention is paid to the quality of the source material. Based upon many studies, scientists have concluded that forms of CJD other than vCJD do not appear to be associated with the consumption of specific foods.

Botulism: Rarer, But Still An Important Concern

Botulism is caused by a neurotoxin that develops from a spore-forming pathogen called Clostridium botulinum. Improper home canning of meats, fruit, and vegetables is one cause. Although the incidence of botulism is low, the mortality rate is high if not treated immediately and properly.

Onset of symptoms in foodborne botulism is usually 18 to 36 hours after ingestion of the food containing the toxin, although cases have varied from 4 hours to 8 days. Early signs of intoxication consist of exhaustion, weakness, and vertigo, usually followed by double vision and progressive difficulty in speaking and swallowing. Difficulty in breathing, muscle weakness, abdominal distention, and constipation may also be common symptoms. Clinical symptoms of infant botulism consist of constipation that occurs after a period of normal development. This is followed by poor feeding, lethargy, weakness, inability to swallow (including saliva), wail or altered cry, and loss of head control.

Feeding honey to infants is one cause of infant botulism. **Infants under 12 months of age, and preferably children under the age of two, should not be fed honey.**

Antibiotic-Resistant Food Pathogens

Antibiotic resistance is a food safety problem for several reasons. First, antibiotic resistance is increasing to some antibiotics, such as fluoroquinolones and third-generation cephalosporins. These antibiotics are commonly used to treat serious infections caused by bacterial pathogens frequently found in food, such as Salmonella and Campylobacter.

Each year, several million people in the U.S. are infected with Salmonella and Campylobacter, which usually cause diarrhea that lasts about one week. Antibiotics are not recommended for the treatment of most of these diarrheal illnesses, but are used to prevent complications in infants, persons with weakened immune systems, and the elderly. Antibiotics may be life-saving for several thousand people each year who have serious invasive infections, such as bacteremia (infection in the bloodstream) and meningitis (infection of the lining of the brain and spinal cord). Salmonella infections are treated with ampicillin, trimethoprimsulfamethoxazole, fluoroquinolones, or third-generation cephalosporins, but some Salmonella and Campylobacter infections have become resistant to these medicines.

A second reason that antibiotic resistance is a food safety problem is that more people may become ill. Ordinarily, healthy persons who consume a few Salmonella may carry them for a few weeks without having any symptoms, because those few Salmonella are held in check by the normal bacteria in the intestines. However, even a few antibiotic-resistant Salmonella in food can cause illness if the person who consumes the contaminated food then takes an antibiotic for another reason. The antibiotic can kill normal bacteria in the gut, letting a few Salmonella that ordinarily would be unlikely to cause illness take over and cause illness.

A third possible reason that antibiotic resistance is a food safety problem is that the food supply may be a source of antibiotic-resistant genes. Harmless bacteria present in food-producing animals could be resistant, and humans could acquire these bacteria when they eat meat products from these animals. Once ingested, resistant genes from these bacteria could be transferred to bacteria that cause disease. Deciphering the extent to which this contributes to a food safety problem is difficult.

For more information on foodborne pathogens and natural toxins visit:
http://www.cfsan.fda.gov/~mow/intro.html

For more information on consumer food safety in general visit:
http://www.foodsafety.gov
http://www.foodsafety.gov/~lrd/advice.html

For additional food safety considerations for commonly consumed individual foods **see chapter four.**

For an excellent overview of food safety practices and even more information visit: **http://www.fightbac.org**

HACCP: A Major Step Toward Food Safety
The FDA supports and promotes the use of Hazard Analysis Critical Control Point (HACCP) programs, an effective and highly utilized food safety monitoring system that was initially used by NASA. HACCP is based on the prevention of hazardous situations throughout the food industry that can lead to foodborne illness.

HACCP involves seven principles:

- **Analyze hazards.** Potential hazards associated with a food and measures to control those hazards are identified. The hazard could be biological, such as a microbe; chemical, such as a toxin; or physical, such as ground up glass or metal fragments.

- **Identify critical control points.** These are points in a food's production—from its raw state through processing and shipping to consumption by the consumer—at which the potential hazard can be effectively controlled or eliminated. Examples are cooking, cooling, packaging, and metal detection.

- **Establish preventive measures with critical limits for each control point.** For a cooked food, for example, this might include setting the minimum cooking temperature and time required to ensure the elimination of any harmful microbes.

- **Establish procedures to monitor the critical control points.** Such procedures might include determining how and by whom cooking time and temperature should be monitored.
- **Establish corrective actions to be taken when monitoring shows that a critical limit has not been met**—for example, reprocessing or disposing of food if the minimum cooking temperature is not met.
- **Establish procedures to verify that the system is working properly**—for example, testing time-and-temperature recording devices to verify that a cooking unit is working properly.
- **Establish effective recordkeeping to document the HACCP system.** This would include records of hazards and their control methods, the monitoring of safety requirements, and action taken to correct potential problems. Each of these principles must be backed by sound scientific knowledge: for example, published microbiological studies on time and temperature factors for controlling foodborne pathogens.

For more information on HACCP visit:
http://www.cfsan.fda.gov/~lrd/haccp.html

Refrigerated Foods
Given that they have been properly transported and stored, the majority of refrigerated foods are safe for consumption until their "Use By" date. Refrigerators should be kept sanitary and all old food thrown out on a regular basis. In most cases leftovers should not be kept for more than a day or so. Refrigerator temperature should be periodically checked to be sure it is below 40 °F.

Frozen Foods
Frozen food that was properly handled and stored at 0 °F (-18 °C) will remain safe for a long period of time. Only the quality of foods suffers with lengthy freezer storage. Tenderness, flavor, aroma, juiciness, and color of frozen foods can all be affected. The process of freezing foods does not

deplete nutrients, and there is little change in protein value when meats and poultry products are frozen. For more detailed information on freezing and food safety visit **http://www.fsis.usda.gov/Fact_Sheets/Focus_On_ Freezing/index.asp.**

> **For a detailed listing of safe storage methods and storage timeframes for a wide variety of foods, see Appendix A.**

Power Outages
According to the CDC, foods in the fridge and freezer are safe for consumption for up to two hours after a power outage. After that, the risk of bacterial contamination rises and the food should not be consumed.

Transportation of Foods
Refrigerated and frozen foods should be transported from the point of purchase to their destination as quickly as possible and immediately placed into a refrigerator or freezer. In warm climates, or when travel time will exceed one hour, perishable foods should be placed on ice in a freezer bag or cooler. Raw meat, seafood, and poultry should be carefully packaged and kept separate from each other, as well as from other foods, during transport and storage. Improperly packaged foods and those that have been exposed to considerable temperature fluctuations during shipment are more prone to contaminants, pathogens, and spoilage. This is equally true for commercially transported foods.

Thawing
Foods should never be thawed or even stored on the counter, or defrosted in hot water. Food left above 40 °F (unrefrigerated) is not at a safe temperature. Even though the center of a package may still be frozen as it thaws

on the counter, the outer layer of the food is in the "Danger Zone," between 40 and 140 °F—at temperatures where bacteria multiply rapidly.

When defrosting frozen foods, it's best to plan ahead and thaw food in the refrigerator where food will remain at a safe, constant temperature—40 °F or below.

There are three safe ways to defrost food: in the refrigerator, in cold water, and in the microwave.

Refrigerator Thawing

Planning ahead is the key to this method because of the lengthy time involved. A large frozen item such as a turkey requires at least a day (24 hours) for every 5 pounds of weight. Even small amounts of frozen food—such as a pound of ground meat or boneless chicken breasts—require a full day to thaw. When thawing foods in the refrigerator, there are several variables to take into account.

- Some areas of an appliance may keep the food colder than other areas. Food placed in the coldest part will require longer defrosting time.
- Food takes longer to thaw in a refrigerator set at 35 °F than one set at 40 °F.

After thawing in the refrigerator, ground meat and poultry should remain useable for an additional day or two before cooking; red meat, 3 to 5 days. Foods defrosted in the refrigerator can be refrozen without cooking, although there may be some loss of quality.

Cold Water Thawing

This method is faster than refrigerator thawing but requires more attention. The food must be in a leak-proof package or plastic bag. If the bag leaks, bacteria from the air or surrounding environment could be introduced into the food. Also, meat tissue can absorb water like a sponge, resulting in a watery product.

The bag should be submerged in cold tap water, which should be changed every 30 minutes so it continues to thaw. Small packages of meat or poultry—about a pound—may defrost in an hour or less. A 3- to 4-pound package may take 2 to 3 hours. For whole turkeys, estimate about 30 minutes per pound. If thawed completely, the food must be cooked immediately.

Foods thawed by the cold water method should always be cooked before refreezing.

Microwave Thawing

When microwave defrosting food, plan to cook it immediately after thawing because some areas of the food may become warm and begin to cook in the process. Holding partially cooked food is not recommended because any bacteria that is present will not have been destroyed and, indeed, may have reached optimal temperatures for bacteria to grow. Foods thawed in the microwave should be cooked before refreezing.

Additional Food Safety Tips:

- Do not use the same bowl and mixer (or utensil) to mix frosting directly after mixing cake batter made with raw eggs. Thoroughly wash the bowl and beaters or utensil with soap and hot water first.
- Do not use a cup or glass, then rinse it without using soap and put it in a dish rack or on a kitchen towel to dry—bacterial contamination results.
- Do not dry hands with a towel (cloth *or* paper) that has already been used to clean up raw or contaminated foods. Change hand towels and cloths often.
- Wash off can lids before opening.
- Avoid tasting food that contains raw ingredients or tasting food that is being cooked with raw or undercooked ingredients (such as sampling cookie dough made with raw eggs or sampling seafood chowder while it's being cooked to see if it's done).
- Never leave foods out on the counter to marinate.

- Avoid purchasing foods past their "Sell By" date or consuming them past their "Use By" date.
- Sanitize the kitchen sink drain, disposal, and connecting pipe periodically by pouring down the sink a solution of 1 teaspoon of chlorine bleach in 1 quart (about 1 liter) of water or a solution of commercial kitchen cleaning agent made according to product directions.
- Avoid buying or using dented canned goods, which may cause botulism.
- Keep the amount of times a food is frozen and defrosted to a minimum to reduce handling risks.
- Avoid eating fish from waterways that have been treated with chemical pesticides or have been used for dumping.

Chemicals & Treatments

Pesticides

The EPA, FDA, and USDA jointly share the responsibility for regulating pesticides used on foods. The EPA determines the safety and effectiveness of each of these chemicals by reviewing studies, then licenses or registers them for use in strict accordance with label directions. This includes reviewing and reregistering older pesticides. The EPA also establishes tolerance levels for residues on raw and processed foods as well as feed crops. These tolerance levels (the amounts of pesticide residue allowable in food products) are generally set 100 times below the levels that are likely or known to cause harm to people or the environment, with special considerations for vulnerable populations such as infants and children. In addition to these tasks the EPA regulates biotechnology for use in pest management (for more information on this topic visit http://www.epa.gov/pesticides/biopesticides/reg_of_biotech/eparegofbiotech.htm). The FDA and the USDA, on the other hand, are responsible for monitoring the food supply to ensure that pesticide residues do not exceed the allowable levels in the products under their jurisdiction.

Plant foods grown commercially or in home gardens are often subject to the use of pesticides. Unfortunately, surface cleaning, which includes rinsing and scrubbing, will not remove pesticide residues that are absorbed into a growing fruit or vegetable before harvest.[6] Organic foods are produced without the use of most synthetic pesticides and offer a viable alternative for those who want to reduce their risk of exposure.

For more information on pesticides and food,
including additional resource links, visit:
http://envirocancer.cornell.edu/FactSheet/Pesticide/fs24.consumer.cfm
http://www.epa.gov/opp00001/factsheets/securty.htm

Fertilizer
Fertilizers used on crops include chemicals, leaves, wood, grass, animal manure, and human sewage sludge. Each has benefits and deficits. Among them, animal manure and human sewage sludge pose some concern due to the potential for improper or incomplete sterilization. These forms of fertilizer may contain drug residues, viruses, and bacteria as well as heavy metals, industrial compounds, and other contaminants. While the use of human sewage sludge is prohibited in the production of organic food crops, the use of animal manure from any source is not.

Chemicals & Additives
There are thousands of chemicals and additives used in the development of conventionally produced foods. They include synthetic food colors, preservatives, artificial sweeteners, dough conditioners, thickeners, and flavorings. In many cases there are numerous additives in an individual product. For example, gums, breath mints, and candies often account for excessive exposure to combined chemical additives. These products can contain as many as five or more types of sweeteners, including the combination of saccharin and aspartame in products that are not sugar-free. Those who are

---

[6] Master, Edward, U.S. Environmental Protection Agency, "Environmental Exposures During Pregnancy," August 23, 2007, <ftp://ftp.epa.gov/r8/ceh/2007/Master.pdf> (December 12, 2008).

sensitive to aspartame and experience headaches or other physical symptoms following its consumption may not realize they are consuming what is generally considered to be a "sugar-free" or "diet" sweetener in a non-diet product. It is also important to be aware that ingredients can change frequently in products, and reading labels regularly can effectively help us to avoid consuming products that can cause reactions or medication interactions. For an informative overview of the safety of numerous food additives, visit **http://www .cspinet.org/reports/chemcuisine.htm.**

Acrylamide
Acrylamide is a chemical that forms when starchy carbohydrate foods are subjected to high heat. It is reasonably anticipated to be a human carcinogen (a cancer-causing agent).[7] While potato chips have often been the focus of media accounts regarding acrylamide, some brands and types of pretzels and even teething biscuits have had higher levels. Sweet potato chips can also contain excessively high levels of this chemical.[8]

For more information on acrylamide visit:
http:// www.cfsan.fda.gov/~dms/ acryfaq.html

For additional testing data regarding this chemical visit:
http://www.cfsan.fda.gov/~dms/acrydat2.html

Packaging
Various government agencies regulate the safety of food packaging materials, which are considered indirect additives due to the fact that chemicals

---

[7] U.S. Dept. of Health and Human Services, Public Health Service, National Toxicology Program, *Report on Carcinogens*, 11th Edition, December 2004, <http://ntp.niehs.nih.gov/ntp/roc/eleventh/profiles/ s003acry.pdf> (December 12, 2008).
[8] U.S. Food and Drug Administration, CFSAN, "Survey Data on Acrylamide in Food: Individual Food Products," July 2006, <http://www.cfsan.fda.gov/~dms/acrydata.html#u1102> (December 12, 2008).

they may contain can leach into foods. Plastic margarine containers, for example, should not be used in the microwave.

For an excellent overview of food packaging materials visit **http://www.fsis.usda.gov/Fact_Sheets/Meat_Packaging_Materials/index.asp**.

Bisphenol-A (BPA)

Bisphenol A (BPA) is a chemical produced in large quantities for use primarily in the production of polycarbonate plastics and epoxy resins. Human exposure to BPA is widespread. It is mainly acquired through diet. The 2003-2004 National Health and Nutrition Examination Survey (NHANES III) conducted by the Centers for Disease Control and Prevention (CDC) found detectable levels of BPA in 93% of 2517 urine samples from people six years of age and older. The National Toxicology Program (NTP) has some concern for effects on the brain, behavior, and prostate gland in fetuses, infants, and children at current human exposures to BPA. Exposure to BPA can be reduced by doing the following:

- Don't microwave polycarbonate plastic food containers. Polycarbonate is strong and durable, but over time it may break down from overuse at high temperatures.
- Avoid polycarbonate bottles and other containers that have a #7 on the bottom (**see http://www.recyclenow.org/r_plastics.html**), as they contain BPA.
- Reduce your use of canned foods.
- When possible, opt for glass, porcelain, or stainless steel containers, particularly for hot food or liquids.
- Use baby bottles that are BPA free.

Toxic Metals

Toxic metals include arsenic, beryllium, cadmium, hexavalent chromium, lead, and mercury. Food-related concerns have included arsenic in certain drinking waters, lead in ceramic ware, and mercury in seafood. Staying alert to government and media advisories can help reduce the risk of consumption in each of these cases as well as others. Also, gardening directly next to homes built before 1978 should be avoided, as lead may be in the soil from the use of lead-based paint.

The GRAS List

Many individual foods and additives reviewed by the FDA over the years can be found on the agency's GRAS (Generally Regarded As Safe) list. A number of additives that were previously on the list have been removed. Today, food producers are allowed to place a food or additive on the GRAS list without FDA review, as the agency suspended its activities in these areas due to funding issues. For more information on the GRAS list visit **http://www.cfsan.fda.gov/~rdb/opa-gras.html**.

Imported Foods

Countless foods, beverages, additives, and other dietary products in the U.S. are imported from other countries. In fact, nearly 6 million food shipments arrive in the U.S. every year.[9] While in many cases this provides benefits to consumers, there are both public and regulatory concerns about imports being produced with less stringent standards than those set forth in the United States. Further complicating the situation is the fact that only a very small percentage of these imported foods are inspected. Risks become even greater when food products are made with ingredients from several suppliers, such as when apple juice is made with concentrates from four or more different countries. According to the FDA, some country's imports are virtually problem-free on a regular basis, while the imports from other countries, including India, Thailand, China, Korea, and many countries in Africa, require "constant vigilance."[10]

---

[9] Meadows, Michelle, "The FDA and the Fight Against Terrorism," *FDA Consumer,* Jan.-Feb. 2004, <http://www.fda.gov/fdac/features/2004/104_ terror.html> (December 12, 2008).
[10] Snider, Sharon, "From Psyllium Seeds to Stoneware: FDA Ensures Quality of Imports," *FDA Consumer,* March 1991, <http://www.fda.gov/bbs/topics/CONSUMER/CON00013.html> (December 12, 2008).

To improve food safety and be more readily able to track potential foodborne illness outbreaks back to their origin, the FDA requires prior notice of imported food shipments. (The FDA expects to receive about 25,000 of these notices daily.) On September 18, 2008, the FDA also proposed label requirements for refused imported foods due to a practice called "port shopping" in which importers have tried to evade import controls after being denied admission into the United States. When FDA refuses to admit a food into the U.S., the food must be exported or destroyed. But some persons attempt to bring the refused food back into the U.S. in the same condition by shipping it to another U.S. port in hopes that the food will be admitted there. The proposed regulation would require that shipping containers of food barred from entry, and any accompanying documents, be labeled as refused. The label would make it easier for FDA to detect previously-refused food.

The proposed rule implements a provision of the Public Health Security and Bioterrorism Preparedness and Response Act of 2002, which provided the FDA with new authority to protect the nation's food supply. The agency currently has authority to detain any food for up to 30 days for which there is credible evidence that it poses a serious threat to humans or animals. In a number of cases imports are held because their labels are not in English or the accuracy of their labeling is questionable.

To learn more about food importation into the U.S. visit:
http://www.cfsan.fda.gov/~lrd/imports.html

Food Bioterrorism

Together with various governmental agencies including the Department of Homeland Security, the USDA, and the CDC, the FDA has developed and is implementing a detailed counterterrorism program to help protect the U.S. food supply. The program includes adding additional staff, assessing food supply threats, and providing emergency preparedness education both for food service workers and the general public. Specifically, the FDA has enhanced food safety by:

- **Working with industry to reduce threats and contain outbreaks of foodborne illness.** The FDA has issued new industry guidance on security measures, and has encouraged specific additional industry security measures in response to the increased threat level. The guidance will help food producers, warehouses, importers, stores, restaurants, and other food establishments minimize the risk that their food will be subject to terrorism.

- **Increasing risk-based surveillance of domestic and imported food.** The FDA has increased inspections of domestic food facilities and sampling and lab analysis of foods produced both here and abroad.

- **Developing the *PrepNet* food safety network.** With the U.S. Department of Agriculture and other federal agencies, the FDA is designing a safety net that will help prevent and respond to chemical, biological, or radiation contamination of our nation's food supply.

- **Implementing the 2002 Bioterrorism Act.** Under the Bioterrorism Preparedness and Response Act of 2002, the FDA requires all of the more than 400,000 domestic and foreign food facilities to be FDA registered. This allows the FDA to follow through quickly on high-risk situations. In addition to requiring importers to tell the FDA in advance about food shipments, the law improves the FDA's ability to detain suspected food, and requires food companies to keep better records so any contamination can be traced back to its source. The law also strengthens the FDA's authority to detain suspect food and allows for more grants to be distributed to the states to help inspect food facilities.

- **Increasing ability to quickly identify outbreaks of foodborne illness.** The FDA is working with the CDC to ensure that outbreaks or unusual patterns of illness are investigated quickly. More effort is needed in this area.

- **Increasing participation in the first Internet-based food safety system.** As of May 2, 2007, 107 federal, state, and local laboratories in 50 states had joined eLEXNET.[11] This shared electronic data system consolidates and shares microbial food contamination findings among federal, state, and local laboratories.

Field Operations

- **Increasing inspections.** Thanks to increased bioterrorism funding from Congress, FDA has hired over 800 new inspectors and other field personnel to keep watch on imports and other avenues our enemies might try to use to contaminate our food or tamper with other FDA-regulated products. FDA now can conduct 24,000 import inspections a year—double the number from 2002.
- **Upgrading laboratories.** The FDA has upgraded its laboratories to handle the increased number of sample analyses. Lab scientists are developing rapid methods for detecting bacterial and viral food contaminants.
- **Scrutinizing imports.**

Toxicological Research

- **Enhancing research facilities and technologies.** The FDA has developed a Level 3 lab at its National Center for Toxicological Research to safely allow analysis and research on select toxicological agents. The lab will be used to test food samples that may be contaminated by biological, chemical, or radiological means. The center is continuing research to identify and characterize biological warfare agents using technologies involving DNA and proteins.

The number of ports that have an FDA presence more than doubled from about 40 ports in 2001 to about 90 ports by the end of 2002. In addition, the agency increased by more than sixfold the number of food import

---

[11] U.S. Food & Drug Administration, U.S. Department of Agriculture, and U.S. Department of Homeland Security, "Agriculture and Food," p. 248, May 2007, <http://www.dhs.gov/xlibrary/ assets/nipp-ssp-ag-food.pdf> (March 10, 2009).

exams conducted at the border, from 12,000 in fiscal year 2001 to more than 78,000 in fiscal year 2003. The agency has also updated its labs to handle the increased number of food samples that may be contaminated by terrorism. There are more than 90 active FDA research projects on the development of tests and sampling methods to quickly detect contaminated food. A major focus is on developing rapid test kits that can be used to quickly inspect food at ports of entry to the United States.

> For more information on food safety and bioterrorism visit:
> http://www.foodsafety.gov/~fsg/ bioterr.html
> http://www.fda.gov/oc/bioterrorism/role.html

Other Safety-Related Issues

Microwaving

Microwaves are produced inside of microwave ovens by an electron tube called a magnetron. These waves are reflected within the metal interior of the oven where they are absorbed by food. This causes the water molecules in the food to vibrate, producing heat that cooks the food. Foods that are high in water content, like fresh vegetables, cook fastest. The microwave energy is changed to heat as it is absorbed by food, and does not make a food "radioactive" or "contaminated."

Although heat is produced directly in the food, microwave ovens do not cook food from the "inside out." When thick foods are cooked, the outer layers are heated and cooked primarily by microwaves, while the inside is cooked mainly by the conduction of heat from the hot outer layers.

Microwave cooking can be more energy efficient than conventional cooking because foods cook faster and the energy heats only the food, not the whole oven compartment. Microwave cooking does not reduce the nutritional value of foods any more than conventional cooking. In fact, foods cooked in a microwave oven may keep more of their vitamins and minerals, because microwave ovens can cook more quickly and without adding water.

The use of microwave ovens is not recommended for home canning, as they are unlikely to produce or maintain temperatures high enough to kill harmful bacteria. Microwave ovens should be kept clean and their seals should be checked periodically. For more information on microwave ovens and food safety visit: **http://www.fsis.usda.gov/fact_Sheets/Microwave _Ovens_and_Food_Safety/index.asp.**

Labeling & Allergies

Food labels must be carefully read when food allergies are a concern. Approximately 2 percent of adults and about 5 percent of infants and young children in the U.S. suffer from food allergies. Each year, roughly 30,000 individuals require emergency room treatment and 150 die due to allergic reactions to food.[12] The Food Allergen Labeling and Consumer Protection Act of 2004 (FALCPA) was enacted to help improve allergen-related labeling and lessen these statistics. For additional information on the Act visit **http://www.cfsan.fda.gov/~dms/alrgact.html.** Other information on food allergies and labeling can be found at **http://www. foodallergy.org /Advocacy/labeling.html.**

Fat and Chemicals

In mammals, including human beings, fat is a storage site for chemicals and toxins. Since many animals used for food are exposed to hormones, antibiotics, and other chemicals, their fat can contain residues of these substances. Fruits, vegetables, nuts, seeds, and legumes can also harbor chemicals in their fat. These chemicals are transferred to our bodies when we consume foods that contain them, where they may stay for long periods of time.

Fat Replacers

Fat replacers can have a variety of different effects on the human body. For example, Olestra, known under the brand name Olean,® has been linked to affecting the uptake of carotenoids (vitamin A precursors) from foods. Further research is needed in this area.

---

[12] U.S. Food and Drug Administration, "Food Allergen Labeling and Consumer Protection Act of 2004," August 2, 2004, <http://www.cfsan.fda.gov/~dms/alrgact.html> (December 12, 2008).

Cookware, Tableware & Utensils

As noted in chapter one, cookware, tableware, and utensils that are ceramic or are made from aluminum or iron have the potential to cause negative health effects. Unlined copper items also have this potential. DuPont was heavily fined by the EPA for not disclosing pertinent information regarding Perfluorooctanoic Acid (PFOA), a chemical used in the manufacture of Teflon.® Using glass or stainless steel can help to lessen any potential risks with regard to these materials.

Industrial Impact

Food crops can be affected by a variety of industrial factors. For example, acid rain caused by the burning of fossil fuels can deplete nutrients from soil, while factory runoff in lakes, rivers, or streams may taint crops with chemicals, byproducts, or waste. Both conventional and organic crops can be affected. Fortunately, the number of beneficial choice-related variables related to crop growth is increasing. An example is the use of ladybugs as a safe and effective means of ridding crops of detrimental insects, a practice frequently used in organic farming.

The Consumer's Role in Food Safety

As consumers, there are many things we can do to ensure the safety of what we consume. These not only include learning about and practicing food safety, but also staying alert to food recalls, learning about the sources of foods and how they are produced, and even growing a food garden without pesticides. We can even check the Department of Health records for the restaurants we like to frequent to find out how they rate in terms of food safety and cleanliness.

Now let's look at how technological changes impact food development and our health.

Food Technology

Food technology covers a broad spectrum of topics that range from food packaging design to the development of sensors that detect chemical and microbiological contaminants in foods. These include nutrigenetics and nutrigenomics, exciting areas of research that study the relationship between genes and nutrition. Here we look at some of the most frequently asked questions about food technologies:

Type of Technology: Irradiation

Is it Safe?
Yes. The Food and Drug Administration has evaluated the safety of this technology over the last 40 years, has found it to be safe under a variety of conditions, and has approved its use for many foods. Scientific studies have shown that irradiation does not significantly reduce nutritional quality or significantly change food taste, texture, or appearance. Irradiated foods do not become radioactive. Irradiation can produce changes in food similar to changes caused by cooking, but in smaller amounts.

Considerations
Food irradiation is a process in which food products are exposed to a controlled amount of radiant energy to kill harmful bacteria such as E. coli O157:H7, Campylobacter, and Salmonella. It is also used to control insects and parasites, reduce spoilage, and inhibit the ripening and sprouting of fruits and vegetables. Food is packed in containers and moved by conveyer belt into a shielded room. There it is exposed briefly to a radiant-energy source. The amount of energy depends on the food. Energy waves passing through the food break molecular bonds in the DNA of bacteria, other pathogens, and insects. These organisms die or, unable to reproduce, their numbers are held down. Food is left virtually unchanged, but the number of harmful bacteria, parasites, and fungi is reduced and may be eliminated.

Irradiation does not, however, sterilize food and does not necessarily kill all pathogens.

Irradiated foods are not widely available at this time. Various stores, however, have sold irradiated fruits and vegetables since the early 1990s. Irradiated poultry is available in some grocery stores (mainly small, independent markets) and at a limited number of restaurants. On the other hand, some spices sold wholesale in this country are irradiated, which eliminates the need for chemical fumigation to control pests. American astronauts have eaten irradiated foods in space since the early 1970s, and patients with weakened immune systems are sometimes fed irradiated foods to reduce the chances of acquiring a life-threatening infection from food pathogens.

FDA currently requires that irradiated foods include labeling with either the statement "treated with radiation" or "treated by irradiation" and the international symbol for irradiation, the radura, as pictured here:

For more information on irradiation visit:
http://www.ars.usda.gov
http://www.physics.isu.edu/radinf/food.htm

Pennsylvania State University also offers an excellent overview
of irradiated foods at:
http://pubs. cas.psu.edu/freepubs/pdfs/uk109.pdf

Type of Technology: Genetic Modification

Is it Safe? Although advocates for genetic modification proclaim its safety, there are many opponents who feel that insufficient or flawed research has been done regarding its potential negative effects on the environment, the ecology, and humans. The potential for allergic reactions to components of genetically modified foods is also a concern.

Considerations

Also called biotechnology, bioengineering, and genetic engineering, genetic modification of crops and food animals is achieved through a process called recombinant DNA, or gene splicing, which gives food plants and animals desirable traits. A large percentage of foods contain genetically modified ingredients and food animals are often fed feed from biotech crops.

For an excellent overview of genetically modified foods visit:
http://oregonstate.edu/instruct/bi430-fs430/Documents-2004/5A-FOOD%20REG/McGorrin%20430_530_2004_rev.pdf

For additional information visit:
http://www.cfsan.fda.gov/~dms/fdbioeng.html
http:// www.ca.uky.edu/brei/faq.htm

Type of Technology: Food Animal Cloning

Is it Safe? On January 15, 2008 the FDA declared that meat and milk from clones of cattle, swine, and goats, and the offspring of all clones, are as safe to eat as food from conventionally bred animals. A lack of both long-term evidence of safe livestock production and long-term product testing, however, has made a number of consumers and researchers uneasy.

Considerations

While cloning may have benefits, such as increased food production, some of these benefits may have the potential to create other problems. For example, if cows can be cloned that are resistant to developing Bovine Spongiform Encephalopathy (BSE), also known as mad cow disease, they may still be exposed to the cause of BSE and develop other diseases.

239

Type of Technology: Pasteurization

Is it Safe? Yes.

Considerations

Pasteurization is a high-heat process that was developed by chemist Louis Pasteur while researching the cause of beer and wine spoilage. The process was applied first in wine preservation. When milk producers adopted the process, pasteurization eliminated a substantial quantity of foodborne illness. Processes used to pasteurize milk include:

Standard Pasteurization. This type of pasteurization improves the quality of milk and milk products and gives them a longer shelf life by destroying undesirable enzymes and spoilage bacteria. For example, the liquid is heated to 145 °F (63 °C) for at least 30 minutes or at least 161 °F (72 °C) for 15 seconds.

Sometimes higher temperatures are applied for a shorter period of time. The temperatures and times are determined by what is necessary to destroy pathogenic bacteria and other more heat-resistant disease-causing microorganisms that may be found in milk. The liquid is then quickly cooled to 40 °F (4 °C).

Ultrapasteurization. This involves the heating of milk and cream to at least 280° F (138° C) for at least 2 seconds, but because of less stringent packaging, they must be refrigerated. The shelf life of milk is extended 60 to 90 days. After opening, spoilage times for ultrapasteurized products are similar to those of conventionally pasteurized products.

Ultra-High-Temperature (UHT) Pasteurization. This typically involves heating milk or cream to 280 to 302 °F (138 to 150 °C) for 1 or 2 seconds. The milk is then packaged in sterile, hermetically-sealed (airtight) containers and can be stored without refrigeration for up to 90 days. After opening, spoilage times for UHT products are similar to those of conventionally pasteurized products.

Processes used to pasteurize other foods and beverages include:

Flash Pasteurization. This involves a high temperature, short-time (HTST) treatment in which pourable products, such as juices, are heated for 3 to 15 seconds to a temperature that destroys harmful microorganisms. After heating, the product is cooled and packaged. Most drink boxes and pouches use this pasteurization method as it allows extended unrefrigerated storage while providing a safe product.

Steam Pasteurization. This technology uses heat to control or reduce harmful microorganisms in beef. This system passes freshly-slaughtered beef carcasses that are already inspected, washed, and trimmed, through a chamber that exposes the beef to pressurized steam for approximately 6 to 8 seconds. The steam raises the surface temperature of the carcasses to 190 to 200 °F (88 to 93 °C). The carcasses are then cooled with a cold-water spray. This process has proven to be successful in reducing pathogenic bacteria, such as *E. coli* O157:H7, *Salmonella*, and *Listeria*, without the use of any chemicals. Steam pasteurization is used on nearly 50% of U.S. beef.

Irradiation Pasteurization. Foods, such as poultry, red meat, spices, and fruits and vegetables, are subjected to small amounts of gamma rays. This process effectively controls vegetative bacteria and parasitic foodborne pathogens and increases the storage time of foods.

Type of Technology: Fish & Seafood Farming

Is it Safe?
The answer to this question depends on the source of the seafood and the treatments it has undergone. Farmed fish and shrimp from other countries may be treated with antibiotics, antimicrobials, pesticides, and other chemicals

which are not permitted per U.S. regulations. They may also be raised in contaminated water.

Considerations

Most fish and seafood farming is done in other countries, such as Thailand and Costa Rica. Some farm-raised fish, particularly salmon, are fed color-enhancing feed, regardless of where they are produced. Sustainably produced farmed seafood raised in clean water is the best option outside of wild-caught types.

Type of Technology: Nutraceuticals

Is it Safe?

Yes, given that there are no contraindications to the use of a certain food or food derivative for a particular individual.

Considerations

Nutraceuticals are foods or food derivatives that are used in the prevention and treatment of disease. This is a growing market with ongoing research and a wide variety of products. The benefits may be particularly great for those who need alternatives or adjuncts to medications due to side effects.

Portions of this chapter were adapted from
the Foodborne Pathogenic Microorganisms and
Natural Toxins Handbook (The "Bad Bug Book").
For more information visit:
http://www.cfsan.fda.gov/~mow/intro.html

Chapter 10

O rganics are a large and growing part of the food industry. They have also become a preferred choice over conventional foods for an increasing number of health-conscious consumers. From milk, meat, and cereals to fruits, vegetables, and condiments, more organic foods and food-related products are being produced and consumed than ever before. Supermarkets, chain stores, and wholesale clubs now regularly carry organic products, many restaurants have begun offering organic meals, and an increasing number of schools throughout the country now serve organic lunches. There are organic markets, organic stores, and an escalating number of vending machines that carry organic snacks. There are even various airlines offering organic foods and beverages in flight. Yet as organics have grown in number, availability, and popularity, they have also attracted controversy. This is mainly due to issues regarding proposed variations in their production.

Here we look at what the term "organic" means along with answers to a variety of common questions associated with this expanding area of nutrition.

Organics, Defined

Organically produced foods are those that have been grown, handled, and processed according to standards developed and regulated by the USDA as part of its National Organic Program (NOP). NOP regulations require that organic crops be raised without using most conventional pesticides; fertilizers made with synthetic ingredients or sewage sludge; bioengineering (also called genetic engineering or genetic modification); or ionizing radiation (also called irradiation). Animals raised organically must be fed organic feed exclusively and allowed access to the outdoors. They are not permitted to be given growth hormones or antibiotics. The actual NOP standards for crops, livestock, and handling are as follows:

Crop Standards

- Land must have no prohibited substances applied to it for at least 3 years before the harvest of an organic crop.
- Soil fertility and crop nutrients will be managed through tillage and cultivation practices, crop rotations, and cover crops, supplemented with animal and crop waste materials and allowed synthetic materials.
- Crop pests, weeds, and diseases will be controlled primarily through management practices including physical, mechanical, and biological controls. When these practices are not sufficient, a biological, botanical, or synthetic substance approved for use on the USDA's National List of Allowed and Prohibited Substances may be used.
- Preference will be given to the use of organic seeds and other planting stock, but a farmer may use non-organic seeds and planting stock under specified conditions.
- The use of genetic engineering (included in the excluded methods), ionizing radiation, and sewage sludge is prohibited.

Livestock Standards

Livestock standards apply to animals used for meat, milk, eggs, and other animal products represented as organically produced, and they require that:

- Animals for slaughter must be raised under organic management from the last third of gestation, or no later than the second day of life for poultry.
- Producers must feed livestock agricultural feed products that are 100 percent organic, but may also provide livestock with allowed vitamin and mineral supplements.
- Dairy animals must be managed organically for at least 12 months in order for milk or dairy products to be sold, labeled, or represented as organic. (Dairy producers may use land that is transitioning during its third year of transition to organic certification to provide crops and forage

for dairy animals during this 12-month period prior to the sale of dairy products as organic).

- Organically raised animals must not be given hormones to promote growth, or antibiotics for any reason.
- Preventive management practices, including the use of vaccines, must be used to keep animals healthy. Producers must not withhold treatment from a sick or injured animal; however, animals treated with a prohibited medication may not be sold as organic.
- All organically raised animals must have access to the outdoors, including access to pasture for ruminants (e.g., cows, goats, sheep, deer, buffalo). They may be temporarily confined only for reasons of health, safety, the animal's stage of production, or to protect soil or water quality.

Handling Standards

- All non-agricultural ingredients, whether synthetic or non-synthetic, must be included on the National List of Allowed Synthetic and Prohibited Non-Synthetic Substances.
- Handlers must prevent the commingling of organic with non-organic products and protect organic products from contact with prohibited substances.
- In a processed product labeled as "organic," all agricultural ingredients must be organically produced, unless they are not commercially available in organic form.

For additional regulatory information on organics visit:
http://www.ams .usda.gov/NOP/indexIE.htm

Now let's look at common questions about organics.

Q & A

Are Organic Foods More Nutritious Than Conventional Foods?

Yes and no. In a recent study of 236 scientifically valid matched pairs of nutrient measurements from organic and conventional food samples, organic plant-based foods were found, on average, to be more nutritious in terms of their nutrient density for several key nutrients.[1] The pairs were derived from 97 peer-reviewed published studies. This would indicate that at least some organic plant-based foods are in fact more nutritious overall than their conventional counterparts. Also, in specific cases, such as when an organic crop has been grown in soil that is more nutrient dense than that of a conventional crop, when organic fruits or vegetables are fresher than conventional ones, or when conventional foods have undergone chemical treatments or other processes that can affect nutrient content even minimally, it is possible for organic foods to be more nutritious. It is also possible for conventional foods to have more of one or more nutrients than organic foods, though they may also contain residues from pesticides, fungicides, rodenticides, or other chemical treatments.

Are Organic Foods Really That Popular?

According to the Organic Trade Association, U. S. sales of organic foods and beverages have grown from $1 billion in 1990 to an estimated $20 billion in 2007. The market for these goods is projected to reach nearly $23.6 billion in 2008, and grow an average of 18% each year from 2007-2010.

---

[1] Benbrook, Charles, et al., "New Evidence Confirms the Nutritional Superiority of Plant-Based Organic Foods," *State of Science Review,* March 2008, <http://www.organic-center.org/reportfiles/ 5367_ Nutrient_Content_SSR_FINAL_ 2.pdf> (December 12, 2008).

Have There Been Any Studies On Humans Comparing Pesticide Exposure From Conventional Foods With That From Organic Foods?

Yes. A collaborative U.S. research study showed that organic diets significantly lowered children's dietary exposure to organophosphorus pesticides. An abstract and details on the study can be seen at **www.pubmedcentral.nih.gov/articlerender.fcgi?artid=1367841**.

Are Organic Foods Better For Infants And Children Than Conventional Foods?

It's likely, given that their young systems are developing and are therefore more prone to potential problems from pesticide residues.

Which Foods Are Best Eaten Organic?

Those whose conventional counterparts are consistently high in pesticides, namely apples, bell peppers, carrots, celery, cherries, grapes (imported), kale, lettuce, nectarines, peaches, pears, and strawberries.[2]

Which Foods Are Less Important To Eat Organic?

Those that consistently have the lowest amount of pesticides, namely asparagus, avocados, broccoli, cabbage, corn (sweet), eggplant, kiwi, mangos, onions, papaya, pineapple, sweet peas, sweet potatoes, tomatoes, and watermelon.[3]

Do Organic Foods Taste Different Than Conventional Foods?

Not necessarily, though they can. An organic apple, for example, may taste different from a conventional apple if it is a different variety, contains more

---

[2,3] Environmental Working Group, "Shopper's Guide to Pesticides in Produce," March 10, 2009, <http://www.foodnews.org/EWG-shoppers-guide-download-final.pdf> (March 10, 2009).

nutrients, was harvested at an earlier or later time, was washed or prepared differently, or other factors.

Can Organic Crops Be Affected By Treatments Done On Neighboring Conventional Crops?

Yes. Pollen drift from genetically modified crops can contaminate organic crops, as can spray drift from pesticides and other chemicals. Water sources can also be a source of contamination.

Can Organic Foods Cause The Same Foodborne Illnesses That Conventional Foods Can?

Yes.

Are There Any Foods Or Edible Substances That Can't Be Labeled Organic?

National Organic Program standards do not currently exist for fish and seafood, therefore they cannot be certified and labeled under the program. Water and salt also cannot be labeled organic.

Why Are Organic Foods Often More Costly Than Conventional Foods?

One reason is that crop yields from organic farms are often smaller than those from conventional farms. Another reason is that organic production is both time and labor intensive, with a number of crops needing to be weeded and maintained by hand to avoid the use of chemicals. Not all organic foods are more costly than conventional foods, however. When they go on sale, and in some cases even when they don't, many actually cost less than their conventional counterparts. As more consumers purchase organics, their price will likely drop.

How Are Organic Foods Labeled?

The USDA's labeling requirements are based on the percentage of organic ingredients in a product and are categorized as follows:

Agricultural products labeled "100 percent organic" and "organic."
Products labeled as "100 percent organic" must contain (excluding water and salt) only organically produced ingredients and processing aids. Products labeled "organic" must consist of at least 95 percent organically produced ingredients (excluding water and salt). Any remaining product ingredients must consist of nonagricultural substances approved on the National List including specific non-organically produced agricultural products that are not commercially available in organic form. Products meeting the requirements for "100 percent organic" and "organic" may display these terms and the percentage of organic content on their principal display panel. The USDA seal (see below) and the seal or mark of involved certifying agents may appear on product packages and in advertisements. Agricultural products labeled "100 percent organic" and "organic" cannot be produced using excluded methods, sewage sludge, or ionizing radiation.

Processed products labeled "made with organic ingredients."
Processed products that contain at least 70 percent organic ingredients can use the phrase "made with organic ingredients" and list up to three of the organic ingredients or food groups on the principal display panel. For example, soup made with at least 70 percent organic ingredients and only organic vegetables may be labeled either "soup made with organic peas, potatoes, and carrots," or "soup made with organic vegetables." Processed

249

products labeled "made with organic ingredients" cannot be produced using excluded methods, sewage sludge, or ionizing radiation. The percentage of organic content and the certifying agent seal or mark may be used on the principal display panel. However, the USDA seal cannot be used anywhere on the package.

Processed products that contain less than 70 percent organic ingredients. These products cannot use the term organic anywhere on the principal display panel. However, they may identify the specific ingredients that are organically produced on the ingredients statement on the information panel.

Other labeling provisions.
Any product labeled as organic must identify each organically produced ingredient in the ingredient statement on the information panel. The name of the certifying agent of the final product must be displayed on the information panel. The address of the certifying agent of the final product may be displayed on the information panel.

Do All Products That Are 100 Percent Organic Or Contain At Least 95 Percent Organic Ingredients Carry The USDA Organic Seal?

Not necessarily. The use of the seal is voluntary, not required.

Can Alcoholic Beverages Be Labeled Organic?

Yes, as long as they meet ingredient and labeling requirements, which are relatively comparable to those for organic foods.

If A Food Is Labeled "Natural" Does That Mean It's Organic?

No. The terms "natural" and "organic' are not synonymous. While natural foods can be organic and vice-versa, a food labeled with only the word natural should not be assumed to be organic or contain organic ingredients.

What Is Organic Certification?

Organic certification is the process in which USDA accredited state, private, and foreign organizations or persons, referred to as "certifying agents," certify that farms and other operations that produce or handle agricultural products that are intended to be sold, labeled, or represented as "100 percent organic," "organic," or "made with organic ingredients" or food group(s) meet the national standards for production and handling practices for organics.

Who Certifies Organic Foods?

There are currently 95 USDA accredited certifying agents, 55 of which are domestic and 40 of which are foreign. To view a complete list of them visit the USDA website at **www.ams.usda.gov** and look under the general information section on the National Organic Program web page.

Who Needs To Be Certified?

Operations or portions of operations that produce or handle agricultural products that are intended to be sold, labeled, or represented as "100 percent organic," "organic," or "made with organic ingredients" or food group(s).

Is Anyone Exempt From Certification?

Yes. Producers and handling (processing) operations that sell less than $5,000 a year in organic agricultural products. Although exempt from certification, these producers and handlers must abide by the national standards for organic products and may label their products as organic. Handlers include final retailers who:

- do not process or repackage products
- only handle products with less than 70 percent organic ingredients
- process or prepare raw and ready-to-eat food labeled organic on the premises of an establishment
- choose to use the word organic only on the information panel
- handle products that are packaged or otherwise enclosed in a container prior to being received by the operation and remain in the same package

251

When Did Organic Regulation Begin And What Entities And Programs Are Involved?

In 1990 congress passed the Organic Foods Production Act (OFPA), which designated the USDA as the governing body for overseeing all types and phases of organics. In turn, the USDA's Secretary of Agriculture established the National Organic Standards Board (NOSB) in 1992. The board's main mission is to assist the Secretary in developing standards for substances to be used in organic production, though it also advises the Secretary on other aspects of implementing the national organic program. The USDA later established the National Organic Program (NOP), which develops, implements, and administers national production, handling, and labeling standards for organic agricultural products and accredits foreign and domestic certifying agents who inspect organic production and handling operations to certify that they meet USDA standards.

What Have Been Some Of The Major Issues Behind The Controversy Over Organics?

One of the main issues has pertained to allowing synthetic substances to be used on organic crops. These substances are listed on the USDA's National List of Allowed and Prohibited Substances. Another issue has been the allowed use of nonorganically produced seeds, seedlings, and other supplies when organically produced or untreated types are not commercially available. Still another issue has involved regulatory changes in the conversion rules for cattle herds, which would leave loopholes for potential nonorganic treatments (such as the use of chemicals) to be administered to cows that are being organically raised.

Is Organic Farming Better For The Environment?

Yes. It enriches soil rather than damaging it, lessens soil erosion, benefits wildlife, protects beneficial insects, and produces less groundwater pollution and contamination, among other things.

Online Organic Gardening Resources

- Organicgardening.com
- Organicauthority.com
- Gardenersnet.com
- Groworganic.com
- Localharvest.org

Additional Online Organic Resources

- OFRF.org
- Organicconsumers.org
- Organic-center.org
- Theorganicreport.org / OTA.com
  Organic Trade Association
  P.O. Box 547, Greenfield, MA 01302
  413-774-7511

Beyond Organic

Sustainable agriculture and business practices:

- FoodAlliance.org

Organic Seeds & Supplies

Eden Organic Nursery Services (E.O.N.S.)
2021 Southwest 70th Avenue, Unit B-9
Davie, Florida 33317
954-382-8281
www.eonseed.com

USDA National Organic Program
Contact Information
Mark Bradley
Chief Agricultural Marketing Specialist
USDA-AMS-TMP-NOP
1400 Independence Avenue, S.W.
Room 4008-South Building
Washington, DC 20250-0268
202-720-3252
202-205-7808 fax
www.ams.usda.gov/NOP/indexIE.htm

Chapter 11

Our bodies have important nutritional needs at every stage of life from pre-birth through our senior years. These needs tend to change—at certain times minimally and at others dramatically—given our age, gender, activity level, overall health, and other considerations. The basic needs of a healthy newborn child, thirty-year-old female, or sixty-year-old male, for example, are all different, as are the extended needs of a premature child, a pregnant thirty-year-old female, or an acutely ill sixty-year-old male. What's important to realize is that no matter what our nutritional needs are at any given time and how they may vary, they always exist. Being alert to how and when they change and knowing how to best meet them gives us an edge in maintaining good health. Presented here is a basic overview of various nutritional requirements and considerations throughout our life cycle.

Pre-Birth

A baby's ability to meet his or her nutritional needs prior to birth is heavily dependent on the mother's overall health and nutritional status both before and during pregnancy. A lack of proper nutrition on the mother's behalf can directly affect not only the child's initial but long-term health and may result in premature birth, low birth weight, birth defects (both physical and mental), spontaneous abortion, or stillbirth. Having an eating disorder, exercising excessively, or engaging in dieting increases these risks. On the other hand, maintaining a well-balanced diet rich in nutrients helps protect the health of mother and child alike. This is an especially important consideration for women who have chronic diseases such as diabetes, hypertension, or phenylketonuria (PKU), or a history of alcoholism or substance abuse.

Specific nutrients of concern during pregnancy are folate and the fat-soluble vitamins A and D. Inadequate folate intake can result in neural tube defects such as spina bifida (in which the fetal spinal column doesn't close during the first month of pregnancy), while an excess of vitamin A increases the risk of kidney problems and central nervous system abnormalities and an excess of vitamin D can cause mental retardation.[1] Alternately, a lack of vitamin D can lead to tooth and bone problems. Fortunately the body naturally produces vitamin D when exposed to sunlight and other forms of ultraviolet light. Women who can become pregnant or are trying to become pregnant should be sure to get at least 400 mcg (micrograms; also written as µg) of folic acid (the synthetic form of folate) daily.[2] The National Academies of Sciences RDA (Recommended Dietary Allowance) for vitamin A for pregnant women 19 to 50 years of age is 770 mcg per day as preformed vitamin A in foods and supplements with a UL (Tolerable Upper Intake Level) of 3000 mcg; for vitamin D the AI (Adequate Intake) is 5 mcg (200 IU) daily as cholecalciferol in the absence of adequate exposure to sunlight.

From Infancy Through Adolescence

Profound development occurs in the human body from birth through adolescence. Nutritional support is critical during this time. Without it, children become vulnerable to many short- and long-term health-related ailments. This includes foodborne illnesses, which children are more readily and dramatically affected by than adults. For example, E. coli O157:H7 and related bacteria, which can cause a serious condition known as hemolytic uremic syndrome (HUS), also often cause acute kidney failure in children.

Establishing proper eating habits at a young age is also essential. Unfortunately, many parents unknowingly and unintentionally pass poor eating habits down to their children instead. This is usually due to habitual consumption of certain types of packaged foods and fast foods. The negative impact of this situation can be substantial. Just as children who are constantly exposed to second-hand smoke are more likely to experience negative health effects, so too are children who are continually fed a diet that is

[1] Grosvenor, Mary B. and Smolin, Lori A., Nutrition From Science To Life, p. 523. ©2002 Harcourt, Inc. Reproduced with permission of John Wiley and Sons, Inc.
[2] Centers for Disease Control and Prevention, "Folic Acid: Questions and Answers," January 30, 2008, "<http://www.cdc.gov/ncbddd/folicacid/faqs.html> (April 15, 2009).

high in fat, sugar, salt, and chemical additives and low in fiber and nutrients. There is much that not only parents but also caretakers and educators can do to help children establish good nutrition, including providing peaceful and positive eating environments. Forced eating is not beneficial and should be avoided.

One of the most serious nutrition-related health concerns facing today's youth is excess weight gain. Data from two National Health and Nutrition Examination Survey (NHANES) surveys (1976–1980 and 2003–2004) show that the prevalence of overweight is increasing: for children aged 2–5 years, prevalence increased from 5.0% to 13.9%; for those aged 6–11 years, prevalence increased from 6.5% to 18.8%; and for those aged 12–19 years, prevalence increased from 5.0% to 17.4%.[3] According to the Centers for Disease Control the NHANES 2003-2004 estimates suggest that since 1994 overweight in youths has not leveled off or decreased, and is increasing to even higher levels. The 2003-2004 findings for children and adolescents suggest the likelihood of another generation of overweight adults who may be at risk for subsequent overweight and obesity related health conditions.[4]

Here is a brief overview of other nutritional considerations in the stages from infancy to adolescence:

Infants

The calorie, protein, and fat needs of infants are far greater than those for adults. This is due to the fact that an infant's organs and bodily systems are growing and developing at a rapid pace. According to the National Institutes of Health (NIH), children who are younger than 2 years of age should receive up to 50 percent of their calories from fat. The NIH also notes that children should not be fed eggs, citrus fruits (or juices), cow's milk, or honey until after their first birthday, or seafood, peanuts, or tree nuts before

---

[3] Centers for Disease Control and Prevention, "Prevalence of Overweight Among Children and Adolescents: United States, 2003–2004," April 2006, <http://www.cdc.gov/nchs/products/pubs/pubd/hestats/overweight/overwght _child_03.htm> (December 12, 2008).
[4] See footnote 3.

age 2 or 3. This is due to the risk of allergy in each case except for honey (which carries the risk of botulism).

Initial nutritional needs must be met through the consumption of either breast milk or formula. Supplemental nutrients may be needed, though their type and dosage must be carefully regulated by a qualified pediatrician. Vitamin K, necessary for blood clotting, is often given to infants at birth in the form of an injection due to the risk of deficiency.

Breast Milk

Human milk contains water, fatty acids, lactose, vitamins, minerals, amino acids, and other nutrients in ideal amounts for digestion, brain development, and growth. It is the best form of nutrition for infants given that the mother is receiving proper nutrition, does not have a substance abuse problem, does not have a communicable disease that may be transferred to the child (such as HIV), and avoids prescription and over-the-counter drugs that can transfer into breast milk and cause harm.

Formula

Infant formulas are substitutes for human breast milk. They are often made with vegetable oils (e.g., soy, palm, coconut, safflower, sunflower) in order to meet an infant's fat requirements. Commercially available types are regulated by the FDA under the Infant Formula Act to ensure safety and quality, though they are not required to be approved before being marketed. An infant's pediatrician should be consulted with regard to the type of formula the infant receives.

For more information on formula-related topics visit:
http://www.cfsan.fda.gov/~dms/inf-faq.html
http://www. cfsan.fda.gov/~dms/ds-inf.html

Introducing Solid Foods

Solid foods are usually (but not necessarily) introduced in the order shown below,[5] with several weeks adjustment time between different types. Ages of introduction are approximate and can vary between babies. A baby's pediatrician is the best source for advice on when and how often any particular food should be consumed. Cereals should be mixed with formula or breast milk unless otherwise directed. Rice, a common ingredient in infant cereals, has recently been shown to cause a severe form of gastrointestinal inflammation known as food protein-induced enterocolitis syndrome, or FPIES, in some infants.[6]

Age	Food	Frequency
4-6 months	precooked baby cereal	twice a day
	baby juices	between meals
5-6 months	strained single fruits	twice a day
6-7 months	strained vegetables	once a day
7-8 months	strained meats	once a day
	plain yogurt	once a day
	baby juices	between meals
8-9 months	egg yolk, strained	once a day

---

[5] Willis, Judith, "Good Nutrition For The Highchair Set," *FDA Consumer,* January 1992, <http://www.cfsan.fda.gov/~dms/wh-hichr.html> (December 12, 2008).
[6] Mehr, S., Kakakios, A., and Kemp, A.S., "Rice: a common and severe cause of food protein induced enterocolitis syndrome," *Archives of Disease in Childhood,"* March 2009, 94(3):220-3. Epub October 28, 2008.

Toddlers

As infants become toddlers, their nutritional requirements change. For example, their calcium needs generally become greater (toddlers between ages 1 and 3 need 500 milligrams of calcium daily, while infants generally need less).[7] To view the overall recommended nutrient intakes for infants and toddlers (as well as all other age groups) visit **www.iom.edu/Object.File/Master/21/372/0.pdf.** It is also important to consult with a child's pediatrician regarding specific individual requirements.

The physical consumption of food is also an important consideration with this age group. Toddlers should be carefully supervised during meals, especially when finger foods such as meat sticks, hot dogs, carrots, cookies, crackers, biscuits, popcorn, and hard candies are being consumed. Foods should always be eaten in an upright position to help avoid choking. Cookie dough and other foods that contain raw eggs should never be given to children (or anyone else for that matter), as raw eggs can carry Salmonella. They also deplete biotin, an important nutrient, from the body.

Children & Pre-Teens (Tweens)

Once past toddlerhood, most children have the capability to broaden their nutritional horizons. Introducing them to a variety of whole-some, low-allergen foods—most notably fruits, vegetables, and grains—at this stage is likely to enhance their chances of enjoying a full range of foods throughout adulthood. It can also benefit them through many critical stages of development leading up to adulthood. However, two important factors should still be kept in mind. First, overconsumption, especially of foods that are high in fat and sugar, can lead to overweight. This is an important concern given that approximately 15 percent of children and adolescents ages 6 to 19 are overweight—almost double the rate of two and a half decades ago.[8]

---

[7] National Institutes of Health, "Infant and Toddler Nutrition," *Medline Plus,* December 9, 2008, <http://www.nlm.nih.gov/medlineplus/infantandtoddlernutrition.html> (December 12, 2008).

[8] U.S. Food and Drug Administration, "Report of the Working Group on Obesity," *Backgrounder,* March 12, 2004, <http://www.fda.gov/oc/initiatives/obesity/backgrounder.html> (December 12, 2008).

(The NIH provides an excellent interactive education program titled Media-Smart Youth for tweens ages 11 to 13 that focuses on the importance of media awareness, nutrition, and physical activity at **http://www.nichd.nih .gov/msy/**). Second, while the types of foods that can be consumed increases for these age groups, the risk of foodborne illness does as well. For an informative overview of this topic visit **http://www.ers.usda.gov /publications/FoodReview/May2001/FRV24I2f.pdf**.

Calcium intake remains an important dietary concern during these years, especially given the allure to replace calcium-rich foods and beverages (such as milk, cheese, yogurt, soybeans, broccoli, almonds, and fortified products, like orange juice) with sodas, candies, and other generally less nutritious foods and beverages. Unfortunately, fewer than one in ten girls and only one in four boys ages 9 to 13 are at or above their adequate intake of calcium.[9] This lack of calcium has a big impact on bones and teeth.

Teens
Today's teens are faced with a number of stress factors that infringe on nutrition, including hectic schedules, school demands, and peer pressure. As a result, they often consume fast foods or junk foods, skip meals, or both. This can lead to overweight and obesity, which in turn can lead to a host of diseases including diabetes and heart disease. Being overweight or obese is also particularly stressful for teens from a social perspective. These very real health problems affect many youth. From 2003 to 2004 alone approximately 17.4 percent of U.S. tweens and teens between the ages of 12 and 19 were overweight according to the NIH. Both parents and teens can find useful answers and helpful guidance with regard to overweight, dieting, and a number of other teen nutritional issues at **http://win.niddk.nih.gov/ publications/take _charge.htm**.

Anorexia, bulimia, and binge-eating disorders are also serious concerns for this age group. (For an overview on these issues and how to find help

March 12, 2004, <http://www.fda.gov/oc/initiatives/obesity/backgrounder.html> (December 12, 2008).
[9] National Institutes of Health, "Why are the tween and teen years so critical?" *Milk Matters,* n.d., <http://www.nichd.nih.gov/milk/prob/critical.cfm> (December 12, 2008).

visit **http://mentalhealth.samhsa.gov/publications/allpubs/ken98-0047/default.asp**.) Even "fad bulimia," a form of binge-eating and vomiting that is practiced by many teenage college females (as well as some males) to avoid weight gain, can disrupt the body's nutritional balance and may lead to true clinical bulimia.

In addition to these considerations, smoking, drinking, and substance abuse among teens also deplete nutrients and can lead to problems and disease that damage the gastrointestinal tract and affect overall health. A lack of calcium remains one of the most important concerns, as by approximately age 17 ninety percent of the adult bone mass for both males and females is established.[10]

Adulthood

There are many factors that can affect the general nutritional needs of an average healthy adult. Among them are stress, illness, injury, overexertion, lack of sleep, smoking, and alcohol consumption. Each of these can cause our nutrient requirements to rise, inhibit our ability to absorb nutrients, or both. (On the other hand, nutrition can *cause* stress, illness, or other health-related problems.)

Gender is also an important consideration. Males and females (especially pregnant females) have considerably different nutritional needs. They also metabolize various foods, beverages, and substances differently. Here are some of the nutritional differences between the sexes along with some general information about each sex:

Females
• Females need more iron than males until after age 50.[11]

---

[10] See footnote 9.
[11] "Iron," Dietary Reference Intakes for Vitamin A, Vitamin K, Arsenic, Boron, Chromium, Copper, Iodine, Iron, Manganese, Molybdenum, Nickel, Silicon, Vanadium, and Zinc. p. 290. Reprinted with permission from the National Academies Press. Copyright © 2000 National Academy of Sciences.

- Women achieve higher concentrations of alcohol in the blood and become more impaired than men after drinking equivalent amounts.[12]
- Research suggests that women are more susceptible than men to alcohol-related organ damage.[13]
- Even low doses of alcohol can raise the risk of breast cancer in women.[14]
- Cola consumption may contribute to lower bone mineral density in older women, a condition that increases the risk of osteoporosis.[15]
- Women are more prone to osteoporosis.
- Women need less fiber than men (25 grams per day between ages 31-50; 21 grams per day thereafter).[16]
- Low levels of vitamin D can increase older women's risk for hip fracture.
- Women are more likely than men to have eating disorders such as anorexia, bulimia, or binge eating.
- The consumption of grapefruit may pose a breast cancer risk for postmenopausal women.[17]
- In women, diabetes is more common under the age of 65, while in men it is more common over the age of 65.[18]
- The risk of heart disease increases for women over 55.

---

[12] National Institute on Alcohol Abuse and Alcoholism, "Are Women More Vulnerable to Alcohol's Effects?" *Alcohol Alert, No. 46,* December 1999, <http://pubs.niaaa.nih.gov/publications/ aa46.htm> (December 12, 2008).

[13] See footnote 12.

[14] Harvard Medical School, "Good nutrition: should guidelines differ for men and women?" *The Harvard Medical School Family Health Guide,* September 2006, <http://www.health.harvard.edu/ fhg/updates/update0906b.shtml> (December 12, 2008).

[15] Tucker, K.L, et al., "Colas, but not other carbonated beverages, are associated with low bone mineral density in older women: The Framingham Osteoporosis Study," *American Journal of Clinical Nutrition,* Vol. 84, No. 4, 936-942, Oct. 2006, <http://www.ajcn.org/cgi/content/abstract/84/4/936>.

[16] National Institutes of Health, "Bone Health," December, 2004, <http://www.niams.nih.gov/ Health_Info/Bone_Health/Nutrition/other_nutrients.asp> (December 12, 2008).

[17] "Study Links Grapefruit to Postmenopausal Breast Cancer," *CANCER,* Vol. 57, 2007, pp. 321-322. © 2007 American Cancer Society. This material is reproduced with permission of Wiley-Liss, Inc., a subsidiary of John Wiley & Sons, Inc.

[18] Morley, J.E., "Nutrition and the older female: a review," *Journal of the American College of Nutrition,* August 1993, 12(4):337-43, <http://www.ncbi.nlm.nih.gov/pubmed/8409092>. (December 2008).

For information on a wide variety of topics related to
pregnancy and nutrition visit
http://www.cfsan.fda.gov/~dms/wh-preg.html.

Males

- The overall nutritional needs of men are generally greater than those of women.
- Men store iron and generally need less than women.
- Men need more fiber than women (38 grams per day between ages 31-50; 30 grams per day thereafter.)[19]
- The risk of heart disease increases for men over 45.
- Anorexia, bulimia, and binge eating affect men as well as women.
- Osteoporosis poses a significant threat to more than 2 million men in this country. After age 50, 6 percent of all men will experience a hip fracture and 5 percent will experience a vertebral fracture as a result of osteoporosis.[20]
- Consuming too much of the omega-3 fatty acid called alpha-linolenic acid, or ALA (found in flax seed and canola oil) or too much calcium may cause prostate cancer in men.[21]

For more information on men's health and nutrition-related issues visit:
http://www.cdc.gov/family/tips/

---

[19] National Institutes of Health, "Bone Health," December, 2004, <http://www.niams.nih.gov/ Health_Info/Bone/Bone_Health/Nutrition/other_nutrients.asp> (December 12, 2008).
[20] National Institutes of Health, "Osteoporosis," August 2008, <http://www.niams.nih.gov/ Health_Info/Bone/Osteoporosis/men.asp> (December 12, 2008).
[21] Harvard Medical School, "Good nutrition: should guidelines differ for men and women?" *The Harvard Medical School Family Health Guide,* September 2006, <http://www.health.harvard.edu/ fhg/updates/update0906b.shtml> (December 12, 2008).

Older Adults

Aging affects our entire body, including our immune system. Many of the changes that occur happen gradually over time, while others happen more rapidly (or at least appear to). While the age of onset for various changes can vary per individual, there are some general timeframes. For example, age-related macular degeneration, in which sharp central vision begins to deteriorate and reading and other tasks become blurry, often begins after age 60, though we may experience such visual changes earlier or later. Hearing changes begin at about the same time, with approximately 30% of people over 60 and about 33% of those 75 to 84 have a hearing impairment, and about half of those over 85 have hearing loss.[22] Immune system changes generally occur gradually, with those 65 and over being more prone to serious effects from illnesses such as the flu.

The actual rate at which we age and the effects we experience are dependent on a variety of factors including our genetics and how and where we live. Nutrition is a key player. Unfortunately, there are a number of things that can affect our nutritional status as we age, including:

- Decreased appetite (due to medications, depression, or other causes)
- Dental problems (e.g., jaw or tooth pain, ill-fitting dentures)
- Gastrointestinal problems (e.g., lack of hydrochloric acid in the stomach, which is needed to digest food)
- Diseases & Illness
- Injury
- Surgery
- Alcohol consumption
- Chemotherapy (cancer treatment)
- Decreased sense of taste and/or smell
- Quality and quantity of nursing home or caretaker-prepared foods and meals

---

[22] Smith, Suzanna and Gove, Jennifer E., "Physical Changes of Aging," *Publication FCS2085,* n.d., <http://edis.ifas.ufl.edu/HE019> (December 12, 2008).

Tricky Tastebuds

A loss of taste can have quite an effect on nutrition as we age, often pro-moting us to use too much salt or sugar—situations that can promote dia-betes, hypertension, and other health problems. This loss is gradual over the years. At birth, tastebuds cover our entire tongues (we are born with approximately 10,000 of them). At the age of thirty, we have approximately 245 taste buds on each of the tiny elevations (called papilla) on the tongue, but by age 70 this number decreases to about 88.[23] This means that by the time we are elderly we may have half the taste buds we were born with. Given, however, that we practice good oral hygiene and avoid smoking, mouth infections, colds, and nasal problems, our ability to taste can remain relatively sharp.

Vitamin B$_{12}$ Deficiency

Vitamin B$_{12}$ deficiency is a serious concern among the elderly. It is esti-mated to affect 10%-15% of people over the age of 60 and often pre-sents itself as anemia.[24] As noted in chapter eight, excess intake of folate can mask anemia caused by a vitamin B$_{12}$ deficiency, which can lead to irre-versible nerve damage.[25] It is therefore important to make sure that vitamin B$_{12}$ intake is adequate, and, if anemia is present, to confirm that it is not due to a vitamin B$_{12}$ deficiency.

Heightened Risks Of Foodborne Illness

While the risk of acquiring foodborne illnesses increases naturally with age due to changes in the effectiveness of our immune system, it can also be increased by the use of improperly cleaned cookware and utensils, the use of foods and condiments that are past their due dates, and other factors.

---

[23] Goard, L.M., "Sensory Changes," *Senior Series #SS-174-R08,* n.d., <http://ohioline.osu.edu/ss-fact/pdf/0174.pdf> (December 12, 2008).

[24] Baik, H.W. and Russell, R.M., "Vitamin B$_{12}$ deficiency in the elderly," Reprinted with permission from the *Annual Review of Nutrition,* Volume 19, ©1999 by Annual Reviews. www.annualreviews.org.

[25] National Institutes of Health, "Folate," *Dietary Supplement Fact Sheet,* n.d., <http://dietary-supplements.info.nih.gov/factsheets/folate.asp#h9> (December 12, 2008).

This is an important concern both for those living alone and those who have caretakers. Vision, hearing, and memory problems can contribute to this increased risk.

Solutions to Chewing Problems
When eating is difficult due to the inability to chew properly, the following foods can provide tasty, nutritious alternatives:

• soft canned fruits
• baked or steamed fruits and vegetables
• creamed, mashed, or cooked vegetables
• ground meats
• yogurt, pudding
• poached, boiled, or scrambled eggs
• nut butters
• oatmeal or other soft cooked grains
• baby or toddler foods
• blended or pureed foods

To view the recommended nutrient amounts for all ages set by the Food and Nutrition Board of the National Academy of Sciences as part of their system of Dietary Reference Intakes (DRIs) visit:
www.iom.edu/Object.File/Master/21/372/0.pdf

Chapter 12

*F*ood labeling is yet another area that has substantial impact on nutrition. Knowing what ingredients a food contains, which treatments, if any, it has undergone, where it was grown or produced, and what its nutritional value is are important factors in our ability to make informed dietary selections and eat healthier. Most if not all of this information can generally be found on food labels, which are required for the vast majority of fresh and prepared foods and beverages, including meat, poultry, eggs, dairy products (and most food products made with them), breads, cereals, canned and frozen goods, snacks, desserts, and packaged drinks. Nutrition labeling for raw produce (fruits and vegetables) fish, and shellfish, however, is voluntary unless a health claim is made. Where produce is sold, nutritional data and information about waxes or other coatings being used is sometimes available on signs. Dietary supplements are in a different category that falls under the general umbrella of foods, but have separate labeling requirements.

The FDA and USDA each play roles in overseeing food labeling and requiring that labels are informative, truthful, and useful to consumers. The FDA oversees the labeling of virtually all foods other than those that are regulated by the USDA or are exempt from labeling. The FDA also oversees the labeling of wines and wine beverages with less than 7 percent alcohol, and bottled water. The USDA regulates labeling specifically for meat, poultry, and egg products. Both the FDA and the USDA require that labels include the name and address of the food product manufacturer, packer, or distributor.

Small business retailers can receive exemption from product labeling permitted that the firm whose name appears on the label has annual gross sales of food to consumers of not more than $50,000 or has total annual gross sales to consumers of not more than $500,000. For foreign firms importing foods, this exemption is based on the total amount of sales to consumers in the United States. Companies that have less than 100 full-time employees and sell less than 10,000 units of food product in the U.S. in a 12-month period are also exempt given that the product being sold is listed with the FDA's Office of Food Labeling and does not make any health claims.

Other exemptions include:

- Foods served or sold in restaurants, unless a claim is made on a label available to the consumer (e.g., fat-free salad dressing).
- Foods served and sold for immediate consumption (e.g., schools, cafeterias, trains, planes, and retail stores, such as bakeries and delis) where there are facilities for immediate consumption.
- Foods that are not for immediate consumption that are processed and prepared primarily in a retail establishment and not offered for sale outside that establishment (e.g., bakeries, candy stores, and delis).
- Foods that are not for immediate consumption and are not processed or prepared on the premises, but are packaged and portioned at a consumer's request.
- Foods that contain insignificant amounts of all nutrients required to be listed in nutrition labeling (e.g., coffee and most spices).
- Infant formula subject to the Infant Formula Act (for more information visit **www.cfsan.fda.gov/~dms/infguid.html**).
- Dietary supplements of vitamins and minerals not in conventional food form.
- Medical foods.
- Bulk foods for further manufacturing or repacking.
- Raw fruits, vegetables, fish, and shellfish, both in and out of the shell, including refrigerated or iced pasteurized crab meat that is not shelf-stable (covered by a voluntary program for display at the retail level; however, when a claim is made, nutrition information must be displayed by the retailer). Fish sold to consumers under the voluntary program must be packaged at the retail establishment.

- Custom-processed fish and game meat. All game meats may provide nutrition information on labeling.
- Foods in packages with available label space of less than 12 square inches (e.g., a pack of gum), provided that the label provides a means for consumers to obtain nutrition information (e.g., address, phone number). If a claim is made, a nutrition label must be provided in accordance with appropriate regulatory requirements.
- Food sold from bulk containers, provided that nutrition information is provided at the point of sale.
- Outer carton label requirements for shell eggs packed in a carton that has a top lid designed to conform to the shape of the eggs, given that the required information is presented inside the carton lid or in an insert.

The Nutrition Facts Label: An Overview

The information in the main or top section on a Nutrition Facts label (above the vitamin and mineral percentages—see Figure 1 next page), can vary with each food product; it contains product-specific information (serving size, calories, and nutrient information). The bottom part (beginning with the vitamin and mineral percentages on the sample label) contains a footnote with Daily Values (DVs) for 2,000 and 2,500 calorie diets. This footnote provides recommended dietary information for important nutrients, including fats, sodium, and fiber. The footnote is found only on larger packages and does not change from product to product.

The Serving Size

The first item on the Nutrition Facts label is the serving size and the number of servings in the package. Serving sizes are standardized to make it easier to compare similar foods; they are provided in familiar units, such as cups or pieces, followed by the metric amount, e.g., the number of grams (denoted as "g"). The size of the serving on the food package influences the number of calories and all the nutrient amounts listed on the top part of the label. **It is important to pay attention to the serving size, especially how many servings there are in the food package.** In the sample label,

271

one serving of macaroni and cheese equals one cup. If we ate the whole package, we would eat **two** cups. That doubles the calories and other nutrient numbers, including the % Daily Values as shown in the sample label (see Figure 2, page 273).

Nutrition Facts

Serving Size 1 cup (228g)
Servings Per Container 2

Amount Per Serving

Calories 260   Calories from Fat 120

	% Daily Value*
Total Fat 13g	**20%**
Saturated Fat 5g	**25%**
Trans Fat 2g	
Cholesterol 30mg	**10%**
Sodium 660mg	**28%**
Total Carbohydrate 31g	**10%**
Dietary Fiber 0g	**0%**
Sugars 5g	
Protein 5g	

Vitamin A 4%	•	Vitamin C 2%
Calcium 15%	•	Iron 4%

* Percent Daily Values are based on a 2,000 calorie diet. Your Daily Values may be higher or lower depending on your calorie needs:

	Calories:	2,000	2,500
Total Fat	Less than	65g	80g
Sat Fat	Less than	20g	25g
Cholesterol	Less than	300mg	300mg
Sodium	Less than	2.400mg	2,400mg
Total Carbohydrate		300g	375g
Dietary Fiber		25g	30g

Calories per gram:
Fat 9   •   Carbohydrate 4   •   Protein 4

Figure 1. Sample Nutrition Facts Label

Comparison of Single & Double Servings					
	Single Serving	%DV		Double Serving	%DV
Serving Size	**1 cup (228g)**			**2 cups (456g)**	
Calories	**250**			**500**	
Calories from Fat	110			220	
Total Fat	12g	18%		24g	36%
Trans Fat	1.5g			3g	
Saturated Fat	3g	15%		6g	30%
Cholesterol	30mg	10%		60mg	20%
Sodium	470mg	20%		940mg	40%
Total Carbohydrate	31g	10%		62g	20%
Dietary Fiber	0g	0%		0g	0%
Sugars	5g			10g	
Protein	5g			10g	
Vitamin A		4%			8%
Vitamin C		2%			4%
Calcium		20%			40%
Iron		4%			8%

Figure 2. A comparison of single and double servings.

Calories (and Calories from Fat)

Calories provide a measure of how much energy we get from a serving of food. Many Americans consume more calories than they need without meeting recommended intakes for a number of nutrients. Excessive calorie intake is linked to overweight and obesity. The calorie section of a label can help with weight management (e.g., gaining, losing, or maintaining). **The number of servings consumed determines the actual number of calories eaten (the portion amount).** In the example, there are 250 calories in one serving of the macaroni and cheese. There are 110 calories in **one** serving from fat, which means almost half the calories in a single serving come from fat. Two servings (the entire package) provide 500 calories, 220 of which come from fat.

General Guide to Calories
40 Calories is low
100 Calories is moderate
400 Calories or more is high

This is a general reference that can be used for calories when we look at a Nutrition Facts label. This guide is based on a 2,000 calorie diet.

The Nutrients: How Much?

Look at the top of the nutrient section in the sample label (page 272). It shows some key nutrients that impact our health and separates them into two main groups: those we should limit and those we should make sure we get enough of.

Limit These Nutrients

Eating too much fat, saturated fat, *trans* fat, cholesterol, or sodium may increase our risk of certain chronic diseases, like heart disease, some cancers, and high blood pressure. These nutrients should be limited.

Get Enough Of These Nutrients

Eating enough dietary fiber, vitamin A, vitamin C, calcium, and iron can help us maintain or improve our health and help reduce the risk of some diseases and conditions. For example, getting enough calcium may reduce the risk of osteoporosis, a condition that results in brittle bones as we age. Eating a diet high in dietary fiber promotes healthy bowel function. Additionally, a diet rich in fruits, vegetables, and grain products that contain dietary fiber (particularly soluble fiber) that is also low in saturated fat and cholesterol may reduce the risk of heart disease.

Note that the Nutrition Facts label can be used not only to help us *limit* those nutrients we want to cut back on, but also to *increase* those nutrients we need to consume in greater amounts.

Understanding the Footnote on the Bottom of the Nutrition Facts Label

Note the asterisk (*****) used after the heading "% Daily Value" on the Nutrition Facts label (see pages 272, 278). It refers to the Footnote in the lower part of the nutrition label (see below), which tells us "**% DVs are based on a 2,000 calorie diet.**" This statement must appear on all food labels. The remaining information in the full footnote, however, is not required to be on the package if the size of the label is too small. When the full footnote does appear, it will always contain the same information. It does not change from product to product, because it shows recommended dietary advice for all Americans—it is not about a specific food product.

* Percent Daily Values are based on a 2,000 calorie diet. Your Daily Values may be higher or lower depending on your calorie needs.			
	Calories:	2,000	2,500
Total Fat	Less than	65g	80g
Sat Fat	Less than	20g	25g
Cholesterol	Less than	300mg	300mg
Sodium	Less than	2,400mg	2,400mg
Total Carbohydrate		300g	375g
Dietary Fiber		25g	30g

The amounts listed under the 2,000 calorie and 2,500 calorie headings in the footnote (page 275) are the Daily Values (DV) for each nutrient listed and are based on public health experts' advice. DVs are recommended levels of intakes. DVs in the footnote are based on a 2,000 or 2,500 calorie diet. Note how the DVs for some nutrients change, while others (for cholesterol and sodium) remain the same for both calorie amounts.

How the Daily Values Relate to the % DVs

Look at the example below for another way to see how the Daily Values (DVs) relate to the % DVs and dietary guidance. For each nutrient listed there is a DV, a % DV, and dietary advice or a goal. If we follow this dietary advice, we will stay within public health experts' recommended upper or lower limits for the nutrients listed, based on a 2,000 calorie daily diet.

Examples of DVs versus % DVs
Based on a 2,000 Calorie Diet

Nutrient	DV	% DV	Goal
Total Fat	65g	= 100% DV	Less than
Sat Fat	20g	= 100% DV	Less than
Cholesterol	300mg	= 100% DV	Less than
Sodium	2400mg	= 100% DV	Less than
Total Carbohydrate	300g	= 100% DV	At least
Dietary Fiber	25g	= 100% DV	At least

Upper Limit - Eat "Less than"...

The nutrients that have "upper daily limits" are listed first on the footnote of larger labels and on the chart above. Upper limits means it is recommended that we stay below—eat "less than"—the Daily Value nutrient amounts listed per day. For example, the DV for saturated fat is 20g. This amount is 100% DV for this nutrient. The goal or dietary advice is to eat "less than" 20g or 100% DV for the day.

Lower Limit - Eat "At least"...

The DV for dietary fiber, listed at the bottom of the example chart (page 276), is 25g, which is 100% DV. This means it is recommended that we should eat "at least" this amount of dietary fiber per day. The DV for total carbohydrate is 300g, or 100% DV. This amount is recommended for a balanced daily diet that is based on 2,000 calories, but can vary, depending on our daily intake of fat and protein.

Now let's look at the % DVs.

The Percent Daily Value (% DV)

The % Daily Values (% DVs) are based on the Daily Value recommendations for key nutrients, but only for a 2,000 calorie daily diet—not 2,500 calories. While we may not know how many calories we consume in a day, we can still use the % DV as a frame of reference. The % DV helps us determine if a serving of food is high or low in a nutrient. A few nutrients, such as *trans* fat, do not have a % DV.

We do not need to know how to calculate percentages to use the % DV as the label (the % DV) does the math for us. It helps us interpret the numbers (grams and milligrams) by putting them all on the same scale for the day (0-100% DV). The % DV column doesn't add up vertically to 100%. Instead, each nutrient is based on 100% of the daily requirements for that nutrient (for a 2,000 calorie diet). This way we can tell high from low and know which nutrients contribute a lot, or a little, to our **daily** recommended allowance (upper or lower limit).

The following page provides a close-up look at the % DV portion of a nutrition facts label.

% Daily Value*	
Total Fat 12g	**18%**
Saturated Fat 3g	**15%**
Trans Fat 3g	
Cholesterol 30mg	**10%**
Sodium 470mg	**20%**
Total Carbohydrate 31g	**10%**
Dietary Fiber 0g	**0%**
Sugars 5g	
Protein 5g	
Vitamin A	**4%**
Vitamin C	**2%**
Calcium	**20%**
Iron	**4%**

Quick Guide to % DV:

5% DV or less is low and 20% DV or more is high.

This guide tells us that **5% DV or less is low** for all nutrients, those we want to limit (e.g., fat, saturated fat, cholesterol, and sodium), or those that we want to consume in greater amounts (fiber, calcium, etc). As the **Quick Guide** shows, **20% DV or more is high** for all nutrients.

If we consider the amount of total fat in one serving listed on the example label above (18% DV) it does not quite reach the "high" category, though if we ate the whole package (two servings) it would double (to 36%) our daily allowance for total fat. Coming from just one food, that amount would leave us with 64% of our fat allowance (100%-36%=64%) for *all* of the other foods we eat that day, snacks and drinks included.

Using the % DV for:

Comparisons. The % DV also makes it easy to make comparisons between products. We simply need to make sure the serving sizes are similar, especially the weight (e.g., grams, milligrams, ounces) of each product. It's easy to see which foods are higher or lower in nutrients because the serving sizes are generally consistent for similar types of foods, except in a few cases, such as cereals.

Nutrient Content Claims. The % DV can be used to quickly distinguish one claim from another, such as "reduced fat" vs. "light" or "nonfat." Just compare the % DVs for total fat in each food product to see which one is higher or lower in that nutrient—**there is no need to memorize definitions.** This works when comparing all nutrient content claims (e.g., less, light, low, free, more, high).

Dietary Trade-Offs. The % DV can be used to make dietary trade-offs with other foods throughout the day. We don't have to give up a favorite food to eat a healthy diet. When a food we like is high in fat, we can balance it with foods that are low in fat at other times of the day. What is important is to pay attention to how much we eat so that the **total** amount of fat for the day stays below the 100% DV.

Nutrients With a % DV But No Weight Listed

When we look at the % DV on food packages for nutrients with no weight listed, such as calcium, we are able to learn how much one serving contributes to the **total** amount we need per day. Experts advise adult consumers to consume adequate amounts of calcium, that is, 1,000mg or 100% DV in a daily 2,000 calorie diet. This advice is often given in milligrams (mg), but the Nutrition Facts label **only** lists a % DV for calcium. For certain populations, they advise that adolescents (especially girls) consume 1,300mg (130% DV) and post-menopausal women consume 1,200mg (120% DV) of calcium daily. The DV for calcium on food labels is 1,000mg.

It is important not to make assumptions about the amount of calcium in specific food categories. For example, the amount of calcium in milk, whether skim or whole, is generally the same per serving, whereas the amount of calcium in same-size yogurt containers (8 ounces) can vary from 20-45 % DV.

Equivalencies

30% DV = 300mg calcium = one cup of milk

100% DV = 1,000mg calcium

130% DV = 1,300mg calcium

Nutrients Without a % DV: *Trans* Fats, Protein & Sugars
Note that *trans* fat, protein, and sugars do not list a % DV on the Nutrition Facts label.

Trans Fat: Experts could not provide a reference value for *trans* fat nor any other information that FDA believes is sufficient to establish a Daily Value or % DV. Scientific reports link *trans* fat (and saturated fat) with raising blood LDL ("bad") cholesterol levels, both of which increase the risk of coronary heart disease, a leading cause of death in the United States.

Protein: A % DV is required to be listed if a claim is made for protein, such as "high in protein." Otherwise, unless the food is meant for use by infants and children under 4 years old, none is needed. Current scientific evidence indicates that protein intake is not a public health concern for adults and children over 4 years of age.

Sugars: No daily reference value has been established for sugars because no recommendations have been made for the total amount to eat in a day. Keep in mind that the sugars listed on the Nutrition Facts label include naturally occurring sugars (like those found in fruit and milk) as well as those added to a food or drink. Checking the ingredient list often provides specifics on added sugars. For example, consider the two ingredient panels below; one for *plain* yogurt (which has 10g of sugar per serving), the other for *fruit* yogurt (which has a whopping 44g of sugar per serving). Note that no added sugars or sweeteners are in the list of ingredients for the plain yogurt, yet 10g of sugars are listed on the Nutrition Facts label. This is because there are no added sugars in plain yogurt, only naturally occurring sugars (lactose in the milk). Also note the source of added sugar (high fructose corn syrup) in the fruit yogurt. Ingredients are listed in descending order of weight (from most to least).

<u>Plain Yogurt</u> - **contains no added sugars**

INGREDIENTS: CULTURED PASTEURIZED GRADE A NONFAT MILK, WHEY PROTEIN CONCENTRATE, PECTIN, CARRAGEENAN.

<u>Fruit Yogurt</u> - **contains added sugar**

INGREDIENTS: CULTURED GRADE A REDUCED FAT MILK, APPLES, **HIGH FRUCTOSE CORN SYRUP**, CINNAMON, NUTMEG, NATURAL FLAVORS, AND PECTIN. CONTAINS ACTIVE YOGURT AND L. ACIDOPHILUS CULTURES.

Other names for added sugars include: corn syrup, fruit juice concentrate, maltose, dextrose, sucrose, honey, and maple syrup.

To limit nutrients that have no %DV, like *trans* fat and sugars, compare the labels of similar products and choose the food with the lowest amount.

Nutrition Facts labels for products intended for infants and small children

Nutrition Facts labels for foods specifically for children less than 4 years of age do not provide % Daily Values for the macronutrients or footnotes at the bottom regarding the percentage of daily values. Also, foods specifically for children less than 2 years of age must not present information on calories from fat and calories from saturated fat and quantitative amounts for saturated fat, polyunsaturated fat, monounsaturated fat, and cholesterol. In both cases, % Daily Value is declared only for protein, vitamins, and minerals.

Produce Labels

Fruits and vegetables often have stickers with what are referred to as Price Look-Up, or PLU, codes on them that are used for inventory and checkout purposes. PLU codes for conventionally grown produce begin with the numbers 3 or 4, while the code for organic produce begins with the number 9 and the code for genetically modified produce begins with the number 8. **Produce companies are not, however, *required* to label a fruit or vegetable as being genetically modified unless it is significantly different from its conventional counterpart, for example, in terms of its nutritional value or because it was developed with a known allergen.** Stickers can also carry brand names, company logos, and the name of the country from which the produce was derived. To search PLU codes, visit http://www.plucodes.com/.

Label Claims

Health Claims

Health claims describe a relationship between a food, food component, or dietary supplement ingredient and the reduced risk of a disease or health-related condition. Such health claims must be qualified to assure accuracy and non-misleading presentation to consumers. To view a summary of those health claims that have been approved for use on food and dietary supplement labels visit **http://www.cfsan.fda.gov/~dms/flg-6c.html**.

Nutrient Content Claims

Claims such as "low fat" and "cholesterol free" may appear on the front of food packages. They describe the fat content of products and can be used only if products meet standards set by the FDA. Here are some examples:[1]

To be labeled:	A food must have:
Fat free	Less than 0.5 gram (g) fat per RACC* and per labeled serving
Sat fat free	Less than 0.5 g saturated fat and less than 0.5 g *trans* fatty acids per RACC and per labeled serving
Low fat	3 g or less per RACC (and per 50 g if RACC is small)
Reduced/less fat	At least 25% less fat per RACC than an appropriate reference food
Low saturated fat	1 g or less per RACC and 15% or less of calories from saturated fat
Cholesterol free	Less than 2 mg per RACC and per labeled serving

---

[1] U.S. Food and Drug Administration CFSAN, "Appendix A: Definitions of Nutrient Content Claims," *A Food Labeling Guide,* April 2008, <http://www.cfsan.fda.gov/~dms/ 2lg-xa.html> (April 5, 2008).

Low cholesterol	20 mg or less per RACC (and per 50 g of food if RACC is small)
Low sodium	140 mg or less per RACC (and per 50 g if RACC is small)
Sugar free	Less than 0.5 g sugars per RACC and per labeled serving

* Reference Amount Customarily Consumed

Additional Considerations

• "Made with whole grains" doesn't automatically mean a food will be high in fiber or nutrients.

• The claim "Light" or "Lite" can be used if 50% or more of the calories in a food are from fat and the fat is reduced by at least 50% per Reference Amounts Customarily Consumed (RACC). If less than 50% of the calories are from fat, the fat must be reduced by at least 50% or the calories reduced by at least one third per RACC.

• "Light" or "Lite" meals or main dish products must meet the definition for "Low Calorie" or "Low Fat" and be accurately labeled to indicate which definition is met.

Structure/Function Claims

Structure/function claims describe the role of a nutrient or dietary ingredient intended to affect normal structure or function in humans; for example, "calcium builds strong bones." In addition, they may characterize the means by which a nutrient or dietary ingredient acts to maintain such structure or function, for example, "fiber maintains bowel regularity," or "antioxidants maintain cell integrity," or they may directly describe general well-being from consumption of a nutrient or dietary ingredient. Structure/function claims may also describe a benefit related to a nutrient deficiency disease (like vitamin C and scurvy), as long as the statement also tells how widespread such a disease is in the United States. **The manufacturer is responsible for ensuring the accuracy and truthfulness of these claims; they are not pre-approved by FDA but must be truthful and not misleading.** If a dietary supplement label includes such a claim, it must state in a "disclaimer" that FDA has not evaluated the claim. The disclaimer must also state that the dietary supplement product is not intended to "diagnose, treat, cure or prevent any disease," because only a drug can legally make such a claim. Further information regarding structure/function claims can be found in FDA's January 9, 2002 Structure/Function Claims Small Entity Compliance Guide: **http://www.cfsan. fda.gov/~dms/sclmguid.html.**

Labeling Of Food Treatments

Genetically Modified Foods
The labeling of genetically modified foods, also referred to as "bioengineered," "biotech," or "genetically engineered" foods, is not required unless:

- the bioengineered food is significantly different from its traditional counterpart such that the common or usual name no longer adequately describes the new food
- an issue exists for the food or a constituent of the food regarding how the food is used or consequences of its use
- a bioengineered food has a significantly different nutritional property
- a new bioengineered food includes an allergen that consumers would not expect to be present based on the name of the food

Irradiated Foods
In most cases, foods that are irradiated are required to carry the international symbol for irradiation, the radura (Figure 3):

285

Figure 3. The radura, the international symbol for irradiation.

The radura must be on packages if the entire product was irradiated, as well as the phrase,"treated by irradiation" (or "treated with irradiation"). The radura can be any color.

There are exceptions, however. According to the USDA, if irradiated meat, such as irradiated pork sausage, is used in another product, then the ingredients statement must list irradiated pork, but the radura symbol does not have to appear on the package. On another note, restaurants are not required to disclose the use of irradiated products to their customers; however, some voluntarily provide irradiation information on their menus.

Food Colors
A variety of coloring agents are used to enhance the appearance of foods, beverages, and other nutritional products. Some are man-made, others are natural. Of the man-made types many are FD&C colors, meaning that they are approved for use in Foods, Drugs, and Cosmetics. They are derived primarily from coal tar and petroleum.[2]

Natural colorants include those obtained from fruits and vegetables. There are also some unusual ones, including those derived from insects (carmine, cochineal).

---

[2] U.S. Food and Drug Administration, "How Safe Are Color Additives?" Consumer Update, December 10, 2007, <http://www.fda.gov/consumer/updates/coloradditives 121007.html> (December 12, 2008).

Packaging

A variety of chemicals are used to bleach, color, coat, seal, strengthen, and protect product packaging. Many are also used to protect product color and quality. For example, additives such as the antioxidants BHA (butylated hydroxyanisole) and BHT (butylated hydroxytoluene) are frequently added to wax liner bags or other materials used to line interior packages to help preserve freshness. This is common with cereals, crackers, candy bars, gum, and snack foods. In these cases the "additives" are in direct contact with the food and have the potential to transfer into it. Statements such as "BHT has been added to the packaging material to help preserve product freshness" appear in the ingredient panel on a number of packaged foods, as required by law. Behind the scenes BHA may be used in butter to prevent rancidity or in beer to help stabilize foaming, while BHT is generally used in cereals and snack foods.

Order Of Ingredients

Ingredients appear on labels in order from those that exist in the greatest amount to those that exist in the least amount, by weight.

Expiration Dates

The dates stamped on most food products reflect the last day a product should be consumed, not the last day it should be sold or purchased. This is especially important with meat and dairy products due to the possibility of spoilage and bacterial contamination. In many cases the date will be preceded by the words "Use By." Some packaging has date stamps with alternate wording, however, such as "Best When Used By," "Guaranteed Fresh Until Printed Date," or "Sell By," indicating that a product may still be used after the date listed. These phrases are often seen on packages of snack foods such as chips, pretzels, and popcorn.

Date stamps may be located directly on bags, packages, bottles, boxes, cans, lids, or caps, or on flat plastic closures used to seal bags. They may be in ink, or imprinted with or without ink. Some are more difficult to find, such as those that are stamped on or near package seals, creases, or crimping.

Pictures
Just because a food product has pictures of food on its label does not mean that the food pictured is actually in the product.

Tricky Wording
Sometimes words or phrases used to market products can be interpreted in more than one way. The terms "No MSG Added" or "No Added MSG," for example, are frequently used on package labels to indicate that monosodium glutamate, a widely used and controversial flavor enhancer that causes physical and neurological reactions in many people, has not been added. This does not mean there is no MSG in the product, however. Not only may it have been added as a sub-ingredient to one or more ingredients within the product—a situation that frequently occurs when companies obtain ingredients from outside suppliers—but it may also have developed during the manufacturing of one or more of the ingredients. When processing is the cause, some manufacturers denote MSG's existence by placing one or more asterisks after the "No MSG Added" or "No Added MSG" statement and providing an explanation at the bottom of the package. For example, an explanation may read "Except for that which naturally occurs in hydrolyzed corn and soy protein." There is debate as to whether the MSG that develops due to hydrolyzation is actually naturally occurring, as hydrolyzation is a high-heat chemical process. Complicating the situation is the fact that MSG does occur naturally in a number of foods, including tomatoes, mushrooms, and parmesan cheese, though it does so in a form that is bound to each food in nature rather than being added as a separate ingredient or chemically caused to develop during commercial production. While the claim being made when the statements "No MSG Added" or "No Added MSG" are used is simply that no MSG has been added, it tends to be misleading.

Unexpected Ingredients

In some cases, foods contain ingredients we don't expect them to contain, such as when high-sodium broth is added to whole chickens and chicken parts that are generally sold without added broth. Reading entire labels carefully is important in order to avoid ending up with something we don't want.

Multiple Suppliers

Many companies manufacture products with fruits, vegetables, meats, or other ingredients obtained from more than one source, and often from more than one country. This may be noted in the ingredient panel (e.g., made with apples from Chile, Brazil, Argentina, and the U.S.) or may appear in another area on a product. The information may be part of the label or may be stamped on.

Ingredient Changes

Product ingredients often change due to supply and demand, recipe alterations, costs, and quality issues. They may change outright from one specific ingredient to another, such as when carrots are replaced with celery, or they may change amidst themselves, such as when carrots are replaced with another brand of the same type. In the latter case, we may never know any change has been made, except in instances where there is noticeable improvement or a decline in quality. We may also be alerted to a change if we begin to have a reaction to a product that did not previously cause any problem. **Reading labels regularly helps us to avoid consuming products that can cause reactions or medication interactions.** However, this does not guarantee that what is written on the package is exactly what's inside. Production and manufacturing errors can still occur.

Labeling Errors

Food labeling errors are not uncommon. During the 2004-2005 fiscal year alone, over ten percent of food samples tested at the Florida Bureau of

289

Food Laboratories had inaccurate labels.[3] In September 2008, the Government Accountability Office issued a report titled "Food Labeling: FDA Needs to Better Leverage Resources, Improve Oversight, and Effectively Use Available Data to Help Consumers Select Healthy Foods." To view the report visit **http://www.gao.gov/new.items/d08597.pdf**.

Other Issues

Allergens

Food labeling errors are a serious and even life-threatening issue for those with food allergies. The Food Allergen Labeling and Consumer Protection Act of 2004 includes provisions for making major food allergens obvious on food labels. These food allergens include, but are not limited to, milk, eggs, fish (e.g., bass, flounder, or cod), crustacean shellfish (e.g., crab, lobster, or shrimp), tree nuts (e.g., almonds, pecans, or walnuts), wheat, peanuts, and soybeans. The University of Florida provides an excellent overview of food labels and allergens at **http://edis.ifas.ufl.edu/pdffiles/ FY/FY72300.pdf**.

Imports

Mandatory Imported Food Labeling

As of September 30, 2008, mandatory country of origin labeling began being required for packages of unprocessed beef, pork, chicken, and nuts (there are, however, some exemptions and time extensions), a move many consumers feel gives them an opportunity to exercise personal choice and more control over their nutritional health. For example, consumers often prefer local products due to the freshness factor. Many consumers also prefer local products due to concerns about the safety of imported foods.

---

[3] Florida Department of Agriculture and Consumer Services, FY 2004-2005 Annual Report. Division of Food Safety. <http://www.doacs.state.fl.us.>

Dietary Supplements

Dietary supplements are defined, in part, as products (other than tobacco) intended to supplement the diet that bear or contain one or more of the following dietary ingredients:

a. a vitamin
b. a mineral
c. an herb or other botanical
d. an amino acid
e. a dietary substance for use by man to supplement the diet by increasing the total dietary intake
f. a concentrate, metabolite, constituent, extract, or a combination of any ingredient mentioned above

Five statements are required to be made on packages and containers of dietary supplements:

1) the statement of identity (name of the dietary supplement);
2) the net quantity of contents statement (amount of the dietary supplement);
3) the nutrition labeling;
4) the ingredient list; and
5) the name and place of business of the manufacturer, packer, or distributor.

For answers to a wide variety of common questions about
dietary supplements visit:
http://www.cfsan.fda.gov/~dms/ dslg-1.html

For additional dietary supplement information visit:
http:// www.cfsan.fda.gov/~dms/supplmnt.html
http:// www.cfsan.fda.gov/~dms/transfat.html#ds

Learning About Ingredients

Developing an understanding about what goes into the foods and products we consume means venturing beyond the basic map of contents and values provided on nutrition labels to learn about specific ingredients and how they affect our bodies. It means becoming familiar with resources that can be used to decipher what certain ingredients are used for, how they are produced, and what their potential effects on our bodies are. It means taking an active interest in building a solid foundation for our health. And it's not hard to do. In fact, it's relatively easy. While nutrition is science-based and often contains technical wording and detailed information, there is also much credible, user-friendly information available. By applying some well-spent effort we can effectively gain an understanding of the roles ingredients play. We can then make choices based on our own personal knowledge rather than solely on what we read or hear in an ad or read on a label. In effect, we achieve a greater degree of control over our health.

Where To Begin

Reviewing the ingredient panels on the foods and products we consume daily is the best place to start. That way we not only have the opportunity to learn about ingredients that are unfamiliar to us, but also to find out about any potential benefits or negative effects associated with those we are exposed to most often. Using a memo pad or notebook to record the names of ingredients we want to investigate is helpful, as it provides a place for notes and updates and is useful for future reference. Care should be taken when transferring words to ensure accuracy, though it should be kept in mind that there can be spelling errors on labels, such as when bisulfite is spelled bisflute. If we are unable to locate a specific ingredient through the resources we choose, contacting the manufacturer may prove helpful. Some companies provide toll-free numbers or website addresses for consumer inquiries directly on their labels.

The next step is research. Colleges that specialize in nutrition often maintain reliable online databases that contain definitions and other information about ingredients. There are also numerous resource books, including *A Consumer's Dictionary of Food Additives* by Ruth Winter, M.S., that provide comprehensive yet easy-to-read information about both harmful and desirable ingredients found in foods. Evaluating write-ups from more than one source is beneficial; it allows us to compare and verify information. In some instances one source may have more data or facts than another. In other cases, two sources may have identical information that they both retrieved from a third-party source. In any case, we should check for information beyond that which is offered by the manufacturer.

The results of this process are eye-opening. Most of us would never consciously indulge in eating acne medication, crushed insects, animal hormones, food treated with carbon monoxide, or even genetically modified foods. Yet most of us already have, and some of us do every day. When we find out, there is usually a combination of anger, shock, and intrigue, or simply disbelief. On the other hand, some of us place complete trust in food manufacturers and regulatory agencies and believe that whatever exists in food must already be checked out and safe, no matter how odd it seems on the surface. The truth is there are allowable levels of many contaminants permitted in foods. There are also many ingredients that have never been tested for effects when they are combined, and numerous claims made by manufacturers that have not been evaluated by the FDA or other authorities.

Once armed with the knowledge of what is in our foods and how it can affect us, we have the option of continuing to use them or finding others with alternate ingredients. This is when reference sources come in handy, as they allow us to check on specific additives or nutrients prior to purchasing the products that contain them.

What Labels Don't Tell Us
Labels don't disclose many things that can affect our health. They don't tell us about sub-ingredients, such as when a preservative that is *not* listed on a

label is used to maintain the quality of an artificial color that *is* listed. They also don't tell us about any exemptions.

For more information on labeling in general visit:
www.cfsan.fda.gov/label.html

For information on meat and poultry labeling terms visit:
http://www.fsis.usda.gov/fact_Sheets/Meat_&_Poultry_ Labeling_Terms/index.asp

---

Chapter 13

$\mathcal{T}$ he relationship between nutrition and health has long been established. Good nutrition is essential for proper growth and development, helps ward off disease, and promotes health in general, while poor nutrition is associated with a multitude of illnesses, many of which can be life-threatening. The leading causes of death in the U.S. that have a known dietary link are heart disease, cancer, stroke, diabetes, kidney disease (due to diabetes and high blood pressure), hypertension (high blood pressure), high cholesterol, and liver disease and cirrhosis, respectively. Here we look at the role nutrition plays in each.

Heart Disease & High LDL Cholesterol

Heart disease encompasses a variety of abnormal heart conditions including coronary artery disease (CAD), arrhythmias, and heart failure. Diet-related factors often involved with these conditions include diabetes (high blood sugar), high blood cholesterol, high blood pressure, overweight, obesity, and the consumption of alcohol. Diets high in fat, salt, and sugar and low in fiber are associated with an increased incidence of heart disease. Diets low in fat, salt, and sugar, and high in whole grains, fruits, and vegetables are associated with a decreased risk.

What does high cholesterol have to do with heart disease?

Cholesterol is a waxy substance found in all parts of the body. When there is too much cholesterol in the blood, cholesterol can build up on the walls of our arteries and cause blood clots. Cholesterol can clog our arteries and keep our heart from getting the blood it needs. This can cause a heart attack. There are two types of cholesterol:

Low-density lipoprotein (LDL) is often called the "bad" type of choles-terol because it can clog the arteries that carry blood to the heart. For LDL, lower blood test numbers are better.

High-density lipoprotein (HDL) is known as "good" cholesterol because it takes the bad cholesterol out of the blood and keeps it from building up in our arteries. For HDL, higher blood test numbers are better.

An easy way to recall which type of cholesterol we want in our blood and which type we don't is to let the "H" at the beginning of HDL cholesterol stand for HAVE foods that promote it in our diet, and the "L" at the be-ginning of LDL cholesterol stand for LOSE foods that promote it from our diet. It is important to note that when total cholesterol levels are high, it may be due to elevated HDL, or "good cholesterol" levels, and not LDL or "bad cholesterol" levels. Checking blood test results carefully can confirm if this is the case.

All adults age 20 and older should have their blood cholesterol and triglyceride levels checked at least once every 5 years.

What do cholesterol and triglyceride numbers mean?

Total cholesterol level - Lower is better. Less than 200 mg/dL is best.

Total Cholesterol Level	Category
Less than 200 mg/dL	Desirable
200 - 239 mg/dL	Borderline high
240 mg/dL and above	High

LDL (bad) cholesterol - Lower is better. Less than 100 mg/dL is best.

LDL Cholesterol Level	Category
Less than 100 mg/dL	Optimal
100-129 mg/dL	Near optimal/above optimal
130-159 mg/dL	Borderline high
160-189 mg/dL	High
190 mg/dL and above	Very high

HDL (good) cholesterol - Higher is better. More than 60 mg/dL is best.

Triglyceride levels - Lower is better. Less than 150mg/dL is best.

We can lower cholesterol through diet by:

Maintaining a healthy weight. If we are overweight, losing weight can help lower our total cholesterol and LDL ("bad cholesterol") levels.

Eating better. Eating foods low in saturated fats, trans fats, and cholesterol.

Eating more:

- Fish, poultry (chicken, turkey—breast meat or drumstick is best), and lean meats (round, sirloin, loin). Broil, bake, roast, or poach foods. Remove the fat and skin before eating.
- Skim (fat-free) or low-fat (1%) milk and cheeses, and low-fat or nonfat yogurt.
- Fruits and vegetables (try for 5 a day).
- Cereals, breads, rice, and pasta made from whole grains (such as "whole-wheat" or "whole-grain" bread and pasta, rye bread, brown rice, and oatmeal).

Eating less:

Organ meats (liver, kidney, brains)
Egg yolks
Fats (butter, lard) and high-cholesterol oils
Packaged and processed foods

Other Considerations
Many of the dietary suggestions for heart disease, stroke, high blood pressure, and diabetes are also applicable for preventing or reducing high LDL or "bad" cholesterol, and vice-versa. For example, the recommendation to consume oats, which are heralded for their heart health benefits and their ability to help stabilize blood sugar, can also be useful in maintaining or improving healthy cholesterol levels. Psyllium seed husk is also known to help reduce LDL cholesterol, and grapefruit pectin has shown potential in reducing it as well.[1]

Diet is not the only precipitating factor in high cholesterol. Age, gender, heredity, weight, our level of physical activity, and stress all affect cholesterol levels too. The National Institutes of Health provides a comprehensive approach to cholesterol management that includes a variety of dietary considerations in its publication titled *Your Guide To Lowering Your Cholesterol With TLC (Therapeutic Lifestyle Changes)*. The complete brochure can be viewed free online at **www.nhlbi.nih.gov/health/public/heart/chol/chol_tlc.pdf**.

Cancer
The link between diet and cancer is highly researched. A number of foods, additives, and toxins are either known human carcinogens (cancer-causing agents) or reasonably anticipated to be. They include ethanol in alcoholic beverages, acrylamide that forms when starchy carbohydrate foods are subjected to high heat, and coal tars from which various food colors and other additives are derived. They also include heterocyclic amines, which form during the cooking of meat, fish, and a number of fried foods, including fried eggs.[2] Overall, diet is estimated to be a causative factor in about one third of preventable cancers.[3]

[1] Bennett, William G. and Cerda, James J., "Dietary Fiber: Fact and Fiction," *Digestive Diseases,* 1996;14:43-58. © S. Karger AG, Basel.
[2] National Institutes of Health, "Factsheet: 11th Report on Carcinogens," January 31, 2005, <http://ntp.niehs.nih.gov/files/11thROC_factsheet_1-31-05.pdf > (June 7, 2006).
[3] Centers for Disease Control and Prevention, "Cancer Fact Sheet," August 30, 2002, <http://www.atsdr.cdc.gov/com/cancer-fs.html> (December 11, 2008).

On the other hand, certain foods are an effective instrumental tool in the fight against many types of cancer. As a whole, fruits provide more cancer-fighting agents than any other food group, though many vegetables do as well. Beans, berries (particularly strawberries, raspberries, and blueberries), cruciferous vegetables (broccoli, cauliflower, cabbage, kale), dark green leafy vegetables, flaxseed, garlic, onions, grapes, green tea, soy, and tomatoes are among the foods that have also shown promise in reducing the risk of cancer.[4] Irradiated products may offer select benefits to those who have cancer and are undergoing chemotherapy, or those who otherwise have compromised immune systems, as they have little or no potential to cause pathogen-related illness.

For more information on cancer and nutrition visit:
http://www.cancer.gov/cancerinfo/pdq/supportivecare/nutrition
http:// www.niehs.nih.gov/roc/toc10.html

Additional information can also be found at **http://www.cancer.org**

Stroke

According to the American Stroke Association (ASA), the following diet-related factors increase the risk of stroke:

High blood pressure — High blood pressure is the most important controllable risk factor for stroke. Many people believe the effective treatment of high blood pressure is a key reason for the accelerated decline in the death rates from stroke.

Diabetes mellitus — Diabetes is an independent risk factor for stroke. Many people with diabetes also have high blood pressure, high blood cholesterol, and are overweight. This increases their risk even more. While

---

[4] Stanford Prevention Research Center and YMCA, "11 Cancer Fighting Foods," n.d., <http://lslw.stanford.edu/11Foods.html> (December 12, 2008).

diabetes is treatable, the presence of the disease still increases our risk of stroke.

Carotid or other artery disease — The carotid arteries in our neck supply blood to our brain. A carotid artery narrowed by fatty deposits from atherosclerosis (plaque buildups in artery walls) may become blocked by a blood clot. Carotid artery disease is also called carotid artery stenosis.

Peripheral artery disease is the narrowing of blood vessels carrying blood to leg and arm muscles. It's caused by fatty buildups of plaque in artery walls. People with peripheral artery disease have a higher risk of carotid artery disease, which raises their risk of stroke.

Other heart disease — People with coronary heart disease or heart failure have a higher risk of stroke than those with hearts that work normally. Dilated cardiomyopathy (an enlarged heart), heart valve disease and some types of congenital heart defects also raise the risk of stroke.

High blood cholesterol — People with high blood cholesterol have an increased risk for stroke. Also, it appears that low HDL ("good") cholesterol is a risk factor for stroke in men, but more data are needed to verify its effect in women.

Poor diet — Diets high in saturated fat, trans fat and cholesterol can raise blood cholesterol levels. Diets high in sodium (salt) can contribute to increased blood pressure. Diets with excess calories can contribute to obesity.

Alcohol abuse — Alcohol abuse can lead to multiple medical complications, including stroke. For those who consume alcohol, a recommendation of no more than two drinks per day for men and no more than one drink per day for nonpregnant women best reflects the state of the science for alcohol and stroke risk.

The ASA also notes that a diet containing five or more servings of fruits and vegetables per day may reduce the risk of stroke. Poor nutritional status early after stroke is associated with reduced survival, lessened functional ability, and altered living circumstances six months later.[5] Therefore proper nutritional support after stroke is essential.

Diabetes

According to the American Diabetes Association, there are 23.6 million children and adults in the United States, or 8% of the population, who have diabetes. While an estimated 17.9 million people have been diagnosed with it, an additional 5.7 million people (or nearly one quarter) are unaware that they have the disease. Another 57 million have pre-diabetes.[6]

Although the cause of diabetes has yet to be discovered, proper nutrition is essential in the prevention of the type 2 form of the disease (also called adult-onset diabetes—though children and teens are now being affected too) and the management of both type 1 (also called juvenile-onset diabetes) and type 2. Harvard University offers the following dietary tips for preventing type 2 diabetes:

Choose healthy fats. A diet rich in mono and polyunsaturated fats can help lower our risk of both diabetes and heart disease. Canola oil and olive oil are great choices, as are the fats in avocados, nuts, and seeds.

Focus on plant foods. A diet high in whole grains can help lower the risk of diabetes and keep our appetite in check. Choose a good variety of whole grain foods prepared in interesting ways.

---

[5] American Stroke Association, "Poor Nutritional Status on Admission Predicts Poor Outcomes After Stroke: Observational Data From the FOOD Trial," *Stroke*, May 15, 2003; 34:1450. www.stroke association.org. Copyright © 2003 American Heart Association. Source: American Heart Association.
[6] Copyright © 2009 American Diabetes Association. From http://www.diabetes.org. Modified with permission from *The American Diabetes Association*.

Cut back on refined carbohydrates and sugary drinks. White bread, white rice, white pasta, and potatoes cause fast and furious increases in blood sugar, as do sugary soft drinks, fruit punch, and fruit juice. Over time, eating lots of these refined carbohydrates and sugar may increase our risk of type 2 diabetes. To lower the risk, switch to whole grains and skip the sugar.

For more information on diabetes visit the American Diabetes Association at **www.diabetes.org**.

Kidney Disease

According to the National Kidney Foundation, the two leading causes of kidney failure (also called end stage kidney disease or ESRD) in the U.S. are diabetes (also called Type 2, or adult onset diabetes) and high blood pressure. When these two diseases are controlled, the associated kidney disease can often be prevented or slowed down. For more information see this chapter's sections on diabetes and high blood pressure and visit **www.kidney.org**.

High Blood Pressure (Hypertension)

In many cases the cause of high blood pressure is unknown. A relatively small percentage is attributed to kidney disease (though high blood pressure can also *cause* kidney disease). Nutritional factors that may increase the risk of developing high blood pressure include overweight, obesity, diabetes, and heavy alcohol consumption. Eating foods that are low in fat and sodium, keeping our alcohol consumption low, and watching our overall calorie intake may help us to prevent developing this common disorder. Avoiding foods that are high in sodium can also be helpful. High sodium foods include most soups (and many other canned and packaged foods), bullions, gravies, soy sauces, and snack foods as well as foods that contain baking soda, baking powder, or monosodium glutamate (MSG). Some meat tenderizers (e.g., Accent), toothpastes, and many antacids also contain high amounts of sodium, as often does drinking water that has been treated. Healthy adults should consume less than 2300 mg (about 1 teaspoon) of

302

sodium per day. The following guidelines are used to label foods for sodium content:

Sodium

Sodium-free: less than 5 milligrams (mg) per serving.

Very low sodium: 35 mg or less per serving or, if the serving is 30 grams (g) or less or 2 tablespoons or less, 35 mg or less per 50 g of the food.

Low-sodium: 140 mg or less per serving or, if the serving is 30 g or less or 2 tablespoons or less, 140 mg or less per 50 g of the food.

Light in sodium: at least 50 percent less sodium per serving than average reference amount for same food with no sodium reduction.

Lightly salted: at least 50 percent less sodium per serving than reference amount. (If the food is not "low in sodium," the statement "not a low-sodium food" must appear on the same panel as the "Nutrition Facts" panel.)

Reduced or less sodium: at least 25 percent less per serving than reference food.

Salt (Sodium Chloride)

Salt-free: sodium-free (see above definition).

Unsalted, without added salt, no salt added:
- no salt added during processing, and
- the food it resembles and for which it substitutes is normally processed with salt.

(If the food is not "sodium free," the statement "not a sodium-free food" or "not for control of sodium in the diet" must appear on the same panel as the Nutrition Facts panel.)

Here are some comparisons of sodium content in common foods:[7]

Meats, poultry, fish, and shellfish
Fresh meat, 3 oz. cooked:	Less than 90 mg
Shellfish, 3 oz:	235 to 900 mg
Tuna, canned, 3 oz:	300 mg
Lean ham, 2 slices:	625 mg

Dairy products
*Whole milk, 1 cup:	98 mg
Skim or 1% milk, 1 cup:	110 mg
*Buttermilk (cultured, lowfat), 1 cup:	260 mg
*Swiss cheese, 1 oz:	55 mg
*Cheddar cheese, 1 oz :	175 mg
Low-fat cheese, 1 oz.:	175 mg
*Cottage cheese (regular), 1 cup:	800 mg

Vegetables
Fresh or frozen vegetables and no-salt-added canned (cooked without salt), 1 cup:	Less than 70 mg
Vegetables canned or frozen (without sauce), 1/2 cup:	55-470 mg
Tomato juice, canned, 1 cup:	340-1040 mg

Breads, cereals, rice and pasta
Bread, 1 slice:	95-210 mg
English muffin (whole)	242-248 mg
Ready-to-eat shredded wheat, 1 cup:	5 mg
Cooked cereal (unsalted), 1 cup:	Less than 10 mg

[7] Source: USDA National Nutrient Database for Standard Reference, Release 18; also general product research.

Instant cooked cereal, 1 packet:	139-241 mg
Canned soups, 1 cup:	443-1,300 mg

Convenience foods

Canned and frozen main dishes, 8 oz:	500-1,570 mg

*These foods can also be high in saturated fat, unless low-fat or reduced fat options are purchased.

Liver Disease & Cirrhosis

There are many causes of liver disease and cirrhosis, though only alcohol consumption is nutrition-related. While a balanced, quality diet can potentially stabilize or improve liver disease or even reverse the effects of early stage cirrhosis, the avoidance of alcohol is critical. Even alcoholics without liver disease are often deficient in amino acids, proteins, and numerous nutrients including vitamins A, B_1 (thiamine), B_2 (riboflavin), B_6 (pyridoxine), C, and folic acid due to alcohol's negative effect on nutrient uptake in the body.[8] Dietary changes for those being treated for liver disease and cirrhosis may include a reduction in the consumption of protein or sodium (or both), avoidance of raw shellfish due to the potential for serious bacterial infection, and complete avoidance of alcohol.[9]

For more information on liver disease and cirrhosis visit:
http://digestive.niddk.nih .gov/ddiseases/pubs/cirrhosis/

[8] Lieber, Charles S., "Relationships Between Nutrition, Alcohol Use, and Liver Disease," NIAAA, September 29, 2004, <http://pubs.niaaa.nih.gov/publications/arh27-3/220-231.htm> (December 12, 2008).
[9] National Institutes of Health, NDDIC, "Cirrhosis," *Publication No. 09–1134,* December 2008, <http://digestive.niddk.nih.gov/ddiseases/pubs/cirrhosis/> (December 21, 2008).

Overweight & Obesity

Obesity is one of the country's most prominent health problems. It is associated with a host of diseases and is attributed to between approximately 280,000 and 325,000 deaths annually.[10] It affects not only adults, but also adolescents and children.

For adults, overweight and obesity are determined by calculating what is known as our body mass index, or BMI. This number is calculated using our weight and height. BMI is used because, for most people, it correlates with their amount of body fat (since it does not directly measure body fat, some people, such as athletes and bodybuilders, may obtain a BMI that indicates they are overweight or obese when in actuality they aren't).

- An adult who has a BMI between 25 and 29.9 is considered overweight.
- An adult who has a BMI of 30 or higher is considered obese.

BMIs for children and teens (also called BMI-for-age) are used to designate being "overweight" or "at risk for overweight." These designations take into account normal differences in body fat between boys and girls and differences in body fat at various ages. The CDC provides a free, easy-to-use BMI calculator for adults, teens, and children at **http://www.cdc .gov/nccdphp/dnpa/healthyweight/assessing/bmi/index.htm**.

Obesity is linked to physical, emotional, and social problems. It increases the risk of many diseases and health conditions including:[11]

- Hypertension (high blood pressure)
- Osteoarthritis (a degeneration of cartilage and its underlying bone within a joint)

---

[10] Allison, David B., et al., "Annual Deaths Attributable to Obesity in the United States," *JAMA*, Vol. 282, No. 16, pp. 1530-38. Copyright © 1999 American Medical Association. All rights reserved.
[11] Centers for Disease Control and Prevention, "Overweight and Obesity," October 24, 2008, <http://www.cdc.gov/nccdphp/dnpa/obesity/> (December 12, 2008).

- Dyslipidemia (for example, high LDL cholesterol or high levels of triglycerides)
- Type 2 diabetes
- Coronary heart disease
- Stroke
- Gallbladder disease
- Sleep apnea and respiratory problems
- Gynecological problems (abnormal menses, infertility)
- Some cancers (endometrial, breast, and colon)

Although there is some push to make the food industry responsible for widespread obesity and other effects on health resulting from the consumption of food products, exercising personal responsibility is by far the more effective option. By being aware of what's in foods and learning how to read and understand labels, we can select foods that are most beneficial for our own health.

For more information on overweight and obesity visit
http://www.cdc.gov/nccdphp/dnpa/obesity/index.htm

Common Digestive Diseases & Disorders

Indigestion
Also called dyspepsia, indigestion causes a variety of unpleasant symptoms including abdominal discomfort, bloating, a burning sensation in the upper abdomen, belching, nausea, and even vomiting or reflux of stomach acid into the mouth.

Causes of indigestion include:
- consuming spicy or fried foods
- overeating or eating too fast (or both)
- eating under stress
- smoking
- drinking alcohol
- taking aspirin or other medications that can irritate the stomach
- stress and anxiety
- gastrointestinal illness
- ulcers
- drinking through a straw, which can cause air to get trapped in the stomach

Ulcers

Peptic ulcers are sores that develop on the lining of the stomach or duodenum (the opening to the small intestine). They are a common affliction, affecting one in ten Americans. There are several causes of peptic ulcers, including infection with a bacteria known as Helicobacter pylori (H. pylori), moderate to extended use of common nonsteroidal anti-inflammatory agents (NSAIDs) such as aspirin and ibuprofen, and cancer in the stomach or pancreas. Peptic ulcers are not caused by stress or eating spicy food, as is commonly believed, though these situations can make ulcers worse. A combination of antibiotics and other medications is used to successfully treat H. pylori.

Constipation

Constipation is the inability to have a bowel movement at least three times per week. It is a highly common problem that affects more than 4 million Americans each year, accounting for 2.5 million physician visits and a consumer price tag of approximately $725 million in over-the-counter laxatives.[12] Those most affected are women (especially after childbirth) and people over 65. Common causes of constipation are:

- not enough fiber in the diet
- lack of physical activity (especially in the elderly)
- medications
- milk
- irritable bowel syndrome
- changes in life or routine such as pregnancy, aging, and travel
- abuse of laxatives
- ignoring the urge to have a bowel movement
- dehydration (lack of water)
- specific diseases or conditions, such as stroke (most common)
- problems with the colon and rectum
- problems with intestinal function (chronic idiopathic constipation)

Getting Enough Fiber

Getting enough fiber is essential to avoid constipation. There are two types: soluble and insoluble. Both have important effects on health. The recommended intake for total fiber for adults up to 50 years of age is set at 25 grams per day for women and 38 grams for men or 14 grams for every 1000 calories consumed. For those over 50, the recommended intake is 21 grams for women and 30 grams for men. **It is important to drink sufficient water when consuming fiber—especially dense or dry fiber such as oat bran—or the fiber itself may cause constipation.** High-fiber foods include:

- Whole grains (breads, cereals, pastas, baked goods)
- Pears
- Pistachios

---

[12] National Institutes of Health, NDDIC, "Constipation," *NIH Publication No. 07-2754,* July 2007, <http://digestive.niddk.nih.gov/ddiseases/pubs/constipation/> (December 12, 2008).

- Berries
- Artichokes
- Lentils
- Beans
- Peas
- Oat bran
- Edamame (soybeans)
- Popcorn (preferably air popped)

Gas

Gas is a common occurrence in most people. It is the cause of burping and flatulence. Certain foods, lactose intolerance, swallowing air when drinking (including when using a straw) and eating can all create gas. Products are available to lessen the amount of gas that develops from eating beans and other foods.

Gastroenteritis

Also commonly referred to as the stomach flu, gastroenteritis is not actually a flu at all, but rather an inflammation of the lining of the intestines caused by a virus, bacteria, or parasites. Viral gastroenteritis is the second most common illness in this country. It spreads through contaminated food or water, and contact with infected people. The best prevention is frequent hand washing.

Symptoms of gastroenteritis include diarrhea, abdominal pain, vomiting, headache, fever, and chills. Most people recover without treatment. An important concern with gastroenteritis is the potential for dehydration. It is essential to drink enough fluids to replace what is lost through vomiting and diarrhea. Dehydration is most common in babies, young children, the elderly, and those with compromised immune systems.

Gastroesophageal Reflux Disease (GERD)

Gastroesophageal reflux disease (GERD) is a consistent form of gastro-esophageal reflux (GER), a common, less serious affliction. GER occurs when a valve-type muscle called the lower esophageal sphincter (LES) opens spontaneously, for varying periods of time, or does not close properly, allowing stomach acid and other contents to rise up into the esophagus. GER is also called acid reflux or acid regurgitation. The esophagus is the tube that carries food from the mouth to the stomach.

When acid reflux occurs, food or fluid can be tasted in the back of the mouth. When refluxed stomach acid touches the lining of the esophagus it may cause a burning sensation in the chest or throat (heartburn or acid indigestion). Occasional GER is common and does not necessarily mean one has GERD. Persistent reflux that occurs more than twice a week is considered GERD, and it can eventually lead to more serious health problems.

People of all ages, including infants, can have GERD. While for some the main symptom is frequent heartburn, others (including most children under 12 years of age) experience other symptoms, such as a dry cough, asthma symptoms, or trouble swallowing.

The actual cause of GERD is unknown, though being obese or having a hiatal hernia may promote it.

Common foods that can worsen reflux symptoms include:

- citrus fruits
- chocolate
- drinks with caffeine or alcohol
- fatty and fried foods
- garlic and onions
- mint flavorings
- spicy foods
- tomato-based foods, like spaghetti sauce, salsa, chili, and pizza

Diverticulosis & Diverticulitis

Diverticulosis is a condition in which small pouches develop in the lining of the colon (also often referred to as the large intestine, although it is actually a separate entity). When these pouches, called diverticula, become inflammed due to irritation or infection, the condition is known as diverticulitis.

The cause of diverticular disease is thought to be a low-fiber diet, as it does not appear to exist in countries with high-fiber diets. Attacks of diverticulitis are likely due to bacteria getting trapped in the diverticula. Eating a high-fiber diet, being active, and staying hydrated may help to prevent or lessen the chance of developing diverticulosis.

Irritable Bowel Syndrome (IBS)
Irritable bowel syndrome (IBS) is a functional problem in which the bowel doesn't function properly. It can cause cramping, bloating, gas, diarrhea, or constipation, or any combination of these symptoms. It is not caused by stress, though stress can make it worse.

Foods and drinks that may cause or worsen IBS symptoms include:

- fatty foods, such as french fries
- milk products, like cheese or ice cream
- chocolate
- alcohol
- caffeinated drinks
- carbonated drinks

Inflammatory Bowel Disease (IBD)
Inflammatory bowel disease encompasses various disorders of the bowel including Crohn's disease and ulcerative colitis. While the exact cause of IBD is unknown, it is believed to be related to an abnormal immune system reaction (known as an "autoimmune" response) to normal bacteria in the intestines.

Symptoms of IBD include constipation, diarrhea, cramping, and rectal or gastrointestinal bleeding. Proper nutritional support is important to prevent excessive weight loss. Eating foods that counteract bouts of constipation and diarrhea can be helpful, as can taking liquid nutrients (given there are no contraindications to their use).

Celiac Disease

Celiac disease is an immune system-related digestive disorder that causes damage to the small intestine and interferes with the body's ability to absorb nutrients. Those with celiac disease have an intolerance to gluten (a protein found in wheat, barley, and rye as well as various nutritional supplements, medications, and other products). A number of people with celiac disease also have type 1 diabetes.

Symptoms of celiac disease vary from person to person. Symptoms may occur in the digestive system or in other parts of the body. Digestive symptoms are more common in infants and young children and may include:

- abdominal bloating and pain
- chronic diarrhea
- vomiting
- constipation
- pale, foul-smelling, or fatty stool
- weight loss

Irritability is another common symptom in children. Malabsorption of nutrients during the years when nutrition is critical to a child's normal growth and development can result in additional problems such as failure to thrive (infants), delayed growth, short stature, delayed puberty, and dental enamel defects on permanent teeth.

Adults are less likely to have digestive symptoms and may instead have one or more of the following:

- unexplained iron-deficiency anemia
- fatigue
- bone or joint pain
- arthritis
- bone loss or osteoporosis
- depression or anxiety
- tingling numbness in the hands and feet
- seizures

- missed menstrual periods
- infertility or recurrent miscarriage
- canker sores inside the mouth
- an itchy skin rash called dermatitis herpetiformis

People with celiac disease may have no symptoms but can still develop complications of the disease over time. Long-term complications include malnutrition—which can lead to anemia, osteoporosis, and miscarriage, among other problems—as well as liver diseases and cancers of the intestine. The only treatment is a gluten-free diet.

For more information, support, and helpful tips visit:
http://www. csaceliacs.org

For more information on digestive disorders contact:
International Foundation for
Functional Gastrointestinal Disorders (IFFGD) Inc.
P.O. Box 170864 • Milwaukee, WI 53217
Phone: 888.964.2001 or 414.964.1799
Fax: 414.964.7176
Email: iffgd@iffgd.org /Internet: www.iffgd.org

Now let's take a look at eating disorders.

Eating Disorders

Approximately 10 million females and 1 million males in the U.S. currently have an eating disorder such as anorexia or bulimia, and millions more are afflicted with a binge eating disorder.[13]

Anorexia

Anorexia nervosa is a disorder characterized by excessive weight loss, a relentless pursuit to be thin, unwillingness to maintain a normal or healthy weight, a distortion of body image, an intense fear of gaining weight, a lack of menstruation among affected girls and women, and extremely disturbed eating behavior. It affects both males and females, with one in four pre-adolescent cases occuring in boys. Some people with anorexia lose weight by dieting and exercising excessively; others do so through self-induced vomiting or the misuse of laxatives, diuretics, or enemas.

Anorexia is both a physical and psychological illness. Physical symptoms of the disorder include:

- impaired physical development
- thinning of the bones (osteopenia or osteoporosis)
- brittle hair and nails
- dry and yellowish skin
- growth of fine hair over body (e.g., lanugo)
- mild anemia, and muscle weakness and loss
- severe constipation
- low blood pressure, slowed breathing and pulse
- cardiovascular and neurological complications
- drop in internal body temperature, causing a person to feel cold all the time
- lethargy

[13] National Eating Disorders Association, "Fact Sheet On Eating Disorders," May 2008, <http://www.nationaleatingdisorders.org/uploads/file/in-the-news/NEDA-In-the-News-Fact-Sheet(2).pdf> (January 12, 2009).

Psychological symptoms include depression, anxiety, and obsessive behavior. Substance abuse is also common.

Treating anorexia involves three components:

1. restoring the person to a healthy weight through proper nutrition
2. treating the psychological issues related to the eating disorder
3. reducing or eliminating behaviors or thoughts that lead to disordered eating to prevent relapse

Bulimia

Bulimia nervosa is characterized by recurrent and frequent episodes of eating unusually large amounts of food (e.g., binge-eating), and feeling a lack of control over the eating. This binge-eating is followed by a type of behavior that compensates for the binge, such as purging (e.g., vomiting, excessive use of laxatives or diuretics), fasting, or excessive exercise, or any combination of these three behaviors.

Unlike with anorexia, those with bulimia can fall within the normal range for their age and weight. However, like people with anorexia they often fear gaining weight, want desperately to lose weight, and are intensely unhappy with their body size and shape. Usually, bulimic behavior is done secretly, because it is often accompanied by feelings of disgust or shame (though "fad" bulimia has become popular among groups of individuals at colleges and in other circles). The binging and purging cycle usually repeats several times a week. Similar to anorexia, people with bulimia often have coexisting psychological illnesses, such as depression or anxiety, and may also have substance abuse problems. Many physical conditions associated with bulimia result from the purging aspect of the illness, including electrolyte imbalances, gastrointestinal ailments, and oral and tooth-related problems.

Physical symptoms include:

- chronically inflamed and sore throat
- swollen glands in the neck and below the jaw
- worn tooth enamel and increasingly sensitive and decaying teeth as a result of exposure to stomach acids
- gastroesophageal reflux disorder
- intestinal distress and irritation from laxative abuse
- kidney problems from diuretic abuse
- severe dehydration from purging of fluids

As with anorexia, the treatment of bulimia often involves a combination of options and depends on the needs of the individual. To reduce or eliminate binge and purge behavior, a patient may undergo nutritional counseling and psychotherapy, especially cognitive behavioral therapy (CBT), or be prescribed medication. Proper nutrition must follow to restore overall mental and physical health.

Binge Eating

Binge-eating disorder is characterized by recurrent binge-eating episodes during which a person feels a loss of control over his or her eating. Unlike bulimia, binge-eating episodes are not followed by purging, excessive exercise, or fasting. As a result, people with binge-eating disorder often are overweight or obese. They also experience guilt, shame, or distress, or any combination of these feelings, about the binge-eating, which can lead to more binge-eating.

Obese people with binge-eating disorder often have coexisting psychological illnesses including anxiety, depression, and personality disorders. In addition, links between obesity and cardiovascular disease and hypertension are well documented.

The treatment options for binge-eating disorder are similar to those used to treat bulimia and include establishing a healthy nutritional regime.

Other Common Nutrition-Related Disorders

Food Allergies

Food allergies are abnormal responses to food triggered by the body's immune system. They are believed to affect up to 6 to 8 percent of children under age 3 and up to 4 percent of adults.[14] Allergens can be passed to an infant through the mother's breast milk. Contrary to popular belief, there is no conclusive evidence that breastfeeding prevents a child from developing allergies later in life.

Common food allergies in adults are shellfish (e.g., shrimp, crab, lobster, crayfish), peanuts, tree nuts (e.g., walnuts), fish, and eggs. Common food allergies in children are eggs, milk, peanuts, and tree nuts (allergy to cow's milk is particularly common in infants and young children). Allergies often develop to foods we eat most often. Children may outgrow their allergies.

Peanuts and tree nuts are the leading causes of the potentially deadly allergic reaction known as anaphylaxis.

Food allergies can be exercise induced and may involve the same symptoms as a typical food allergy experienced simply by eating, including itching, hives, and even anaphylaxis. Avoiding exercise within a couple of hours after eating can reduce the risk of a reaction.

Allergies are cross reactive, meaning that foods or other substances in the same family as a known allergen can also cause a reaction. For example, if we are allergic to shrimp, we are generally allergic to all shellfish. This is known as "oral allergy syndrome." Cross reactivity is not only found from among foods. For example, those who are allergic to ragweed are often unable to tolerate eating melon, particularly cantaloupe. Those with a strong birch pollen allergy may react to apple peels. And those with who are highly sensitive to poison oak are likely to react to mangos.

---

[14] National Institutes of Health, "Food Allergy: An Overview," *Publication No. 07-5518,* July 2007, <http://www3.niaid.nih.gov/topics/foodAllergy/PDF/foodallergy.pdf> (December 12, 2008).

Allergies may be detected through an elimination diet, skin test, or blood test. Blood tests available include the RAST (radio-allergosorbent) test and newer ones such as the CAP-RAST. Another blood test is called ELISA (enzyme linked immunosorbent assay). These blood tests measure the presence of food-specific IgE in the blood. The CAP-RAST can measure how much IgE the blood has to a specific food. Positive skin or blood tests do not definitively indicate that a food allergy is present.

For more information on allergies visit:

http://www3.niaid.nih.gov/topics/foodAllergy/PDF/foodallergy.pdf
http://www.foodallergy.org

Food Intolerance
Many people are sensitive or intolerant to certain foods. Gluten intolerance (celiac disease), lactose intolerance (a deficiency of lactase, the enzyme that breaks down lactose found in milk), and sensitivity to food additives such as preservatives, artificial sweeteners, food colors, and monosodium glutamate (MSG) are among the most commonly reported problems. Avoidance is the most effective treatment in most cases, though for lactose intolerance lactase enzyme tablets or capsules can be taken to avoid symptoms.

Hypoglycemia
Hypoglycemia, also called low blood sugar, occurs when our blood glucose (blood sugar) level drops too low to provide enough energy for our body's activities. In adults and children over 10 years of age it is uncommon except as a side effect of diabetes treatment, though it can also result from other medications (including aspirin, quinine, and sulfa), diseases other than diabetes, tumors, and hormone or enzyme deficiencies. Exercise and alcohol consumption can also promote hypoglycemia.

There are two types of hypoglycemia that can occur in those without diabetes: reactive (after meals) and fasting. Reactive hypoglycemia is characterized by an onset of symptoms within four hours after eating. Fasting hypoglycemia is that which can occur upon waking, after heavy exercise, or between meals and is indicated by a blood glucose level of less than 50 mg/dL.

Symptoms of hypoglycemia include:
- hunger
- nervousness and shakiness
- perspiration
- dizziness or light-headedness
- sleepiness
- confusion
- difficulty speaking
- feeling anxious or weak
- nightmares
- feeling tired, irritable, or confused upon waking

The following recommendations may help those who are not diabetic to avoid hypoglycemic episodes:
- eat small meals and snacks about every 3 hours
- exercise regularly and sensibly
- eat a well-balanced diet
- choose high-fiber foods
- avoid or limit foods high in sugar, especially on an empty stomach

Those with diabetes should follow the recommendations of their physician.

Anemia

Iron deficiency is the most common nutritional deficiency in this country.[15] For those who are not affected by the genetic "iron overload" disorder known

---

[15] Centers for Disease Control and Prevention, "Recommendations to Prevent and Control Iron Deficiency in the United States, n.d., <http://www.cdc.gov/mmwr/preview/mmwrhtml/00051880.htm> (December 12, 2008).

as primary hemochromatosis, which can cause iron toxicity, eating a balanced diet that includes iron-rich foods such as lentils, peas, spinach, liver, beef, poultry, salmon, shellfish, whole grains, sunflower seeds, and parsley is the best prevention. Men store iron; women lose iron, therefore a woman's need for iron intake is generally greater than a man's during her childbearing years.

Candidiasis (Yeast Infection)
Candidiasis is an overgrowth of candida (yeast) in the body. It can be caused by illness, hormonal imbalances, the use of antibiotics, and other factors. It can affect many areas of the body, including the mouth, where it is referred to as "thrush," and the esophagus, where it is referred to as "esophagitis." In addition to antifungal medications, the use of Lactobacillus acidophilus and consuming a balanced diet that is low in sugar (including fruit sugar) can be helpful. For information on a variety of helpful topics related to candidiasis visit **http://www.nlm.nih.gov/medlineplus/yeast infections.html#cat3**.

Mental Health
Proper nutrition has a positive impact on mental health, providing benefits that help us to avoid, improve, or alleviate a number of conditions ranging from anxiety and depression to serious functional brain disorders such as Alzheimer's disease. Poor nutrition can have the opposite effect. A lack of niacin (vitamin B3), for instance, can lead to depression or dementia.

Chemical exposure through diet can also have a negative mental impact. For example, the ingestion of lead by young children from tainted food or water (or from foods or beverages stored or served in containers made with lead-based paint) can cause hyperactivity, an inability to focus, or even brain damage. On the whole, eating a well-balanced diet and reducing our exposure to chemicals in foods can help protect and enhance our mental health.

Dental Health

Dental health not only plays a major role in obtaining good nutrition, but is also an important indicator of overall health. The condition of our teeth, gums, and tongue can reveal many things, including what we do and don't eat or drink, if we are short of particular nutrients, if we smoke, if we are bulimic, if we have thrush (which may indicate a weakened immune system), and possibly even the condition of our heart.[16]

On the other hand, practicing proper dental hygiene and keeping our mouths in optimum condition by brushing, flossing, and obtaining regular dental care gives us the ability to chew nutrient-rich foods such as whole grains, seeds, and nuts that can better our health (nut butters, such as cashew butter, are excellent options for those who have difficulty chewing or digesting nuts whole). By maintaining good dental health we can achieve or maintain good overall health, and vice-versa.

Nutrition & Preventive Care

Today, views on medicine and nutrition are coming closer together than ever, and in many cases they are merging. Physicians, medical groups, and other related entities now have nutrition personnel on staff. Many doctors are taking courses on nutrition. And a number of well-recognized and highly respected medical doctors now publicly emphasize the importance of nutrition as part of preventive healthcare. Using nutrition to improve or maintain our health is not a new concept, however, but rather one that is being put into practice more often as critical changes in both the medical and nutritional industries are taking place. It is due in part to the fact that we as consumers have become more conscious about changes in food production and more proactive with regard to our own food-related health issues.

With valid research as a common denominator, unity between different schools of thought on nutrition, including those from both the mainstream

---

[16] Harvard Medical School, "Heart disease and oral health: role of oral bacteria in heart plaque," *Harvard Health Publications,* February 2007, <http://www.health.harvard.edu/press_releases/heart-disease-oral-health.htm> (March 1, 2009).

and alternative sectors, can help us to bridge gaps in understanding how to prevent and manage cancer, diabetes, and other devastating illnesses. It can also help us to further the knowledge that adding enzyme-filled, nutrient-rich foods to a program that includes other healthful regimens is beneficial for the health of mankind.

Chapter 14

Food & Drug Interactions

IMPORTANT NOTE: The following information, which includes recommendations and warnings regarding interactions between food, herbs, and alcohol (or any combination of these) and the use of specific medications, is provided for use as a basic guide only and may not be complete due to updates made after publication or other reasons. This listing does not cover all possible food-drug or drug-drug interactions. Always be sure to check with qualified doctors and pharmacists for complete, current information regarding all medications before use.

Information provided here was developed by Poudre Valley Hospital's Medical Nutrition Therapy Services and Pharmacy Services and is reprinted from the hospital's *Food & Drug Interactions* pamphlet with permission.

Medication	Recommendations & Potential Problems
ANALGESICS	
<u>Aspirin & Nonsteroidal</u> <u>Anti-Inflammatory</u> <u>Drugs (NSAIDs)</u> **Aspirin & Other Salicylates** (Trilisate, Disalcid, Dolobid) **Ibuprofen** (Advil, Motrin, Nuprin, and various other brands) **Ketoprofen** (Orudus KT) **Naproxen** (Aleve, Naprosyn, Anaprox) **Other NSAIDs** (Indocin, Clinoril, Daypro, Feldene, Lodine, Relafen, Toradol, Voltaren, etc.)	These medications may cause stomach upset and should be taken with milk or food. *Do not take these drugs in combination, and do not take with anticoagulants such as Coumadin without discussing risks with your doctor or pharmacist.* Gastrointestinal bleeding may result from improper or excessive use.
Cox-II Inhibitors Rofecoxib (Vioxx), Celecoxib (Celebrex), Valdecoxib (Bextra)	May take with or without food.

Narcotic Analgesics	
Morphine, Codeine, Meperidine (Demerol) **Percocet, Percodan, Tylox, Vicodin, other narcotics**	Cause drowsiness. ***Avoid alcoholic beverages.*** May cause constipation and stomach upset. Take with milk or food.
Phenazopyridine (Pyridium)	Take 1/2 hour before meals with a full glass of water. May change color of urine.

ANTIBIOTICS	
Cephalosporins (Ceclor, Ceftin, Keflex, Velosef)	For best results, take on an empty stomach (1 hour before meals or 2 hours after meals). If stomach irritation occurs, take with milk or light snack, i.e. crackers.
Erythromycins (E-mycin, Erytab, EryC, Biaxin, Zithromax)	May take with food if stomach upset occurs. ***Avoid taking with citrus food, citrus juices, and carbonated drinks.***
Metronidazole (Flagyl)	May cause upset stomach. Take with food ***Avoid alcoholic beverages, as nausea and vomiting may occur.***
Nitrofurantoin (Macrodantin)	May cause stomach upset. For best results take with milk or food. May change color of urine.
Penicillins (PenG, Pentids, Ampicillin)	Take on an empty stomach (1 hour before or 2 hours after meals). Take with a full glass of

	water. *Avoid taking with citrus foods or citrus juices and carbonated beverages.*
Amoxicillin, Pen VK, Augmentin	Absorption unaffected by food.
Linezolid (Zyvox)	*Avoid food high in tyramine* (see *Foods High in Tyramine chart*).
Quinolones (Levaquin, Cipro, Floxin, Noroxin)	*Avoid antacids 2 hours before and 3 hours after taking medication.* Take with a full glass of water.
Tetracycline	*Avoid iron and calcium supplements, antacids, and milk and milk products.* For best results, take on an empty stomach (1 hour before or 2 hours after meals.)
ANTICOAGULANTS	
Warfarin (Coumadin, Dicoumarol)	*Avoid alcoholic beverages, aspirin, aspirin-like products and nonsteroidal anti-inflammatory medicines (NSAIDS) such as Advil, Motrin, and Aleve unless you have checked with your doctor.* *Avoid the following herbal products: Cinnabar Root, Chlorella, Ginger, Garlic, Ginkgo Biloba, Guar Gum, Dong Quai, Feverfew, Ginseng.* Maintain a consistent diet of foods containing Vitamin K. *See Foods High in Vitamin K chart.*

CARDIOVASCULAR DRUGS	
ACE Inhibitors	Take on an empty stomach. *Avoid the herbal product St. John's Wort.*
Nitrates (Isordil, Imdur, Sorbitrate)	*Avoid alcoholic beverages.* Take on an empty stomach (1 hour before or 2 hours after meals).
Digoxin (Lanoxin)	Take oral dose after morning meal. *Avoid antacids; cough, cold, and allergy products; and appetite suppressants. Avoid the herbal products St. John's Wort, Foxglove. Licorice may increase the risk for toxicity of this drug.*
Dipyridamole (Persantine)	Take 1 hour before meals with a full glass of water.
Quinidine (Quinaglute, Quinora)	May cause stomach upset. Take with food.
Diltiazem (Cardizem)	Take before meals. *Avoid the herbal product St. John's Wort.*
DIURETICS	
(See Chart of Foods High In Potassium)	
<u>Potassium Depleting</u>	
Bumetanide (Bumex)	Include high potassium foods in diet.
Furosemide (Lasix)	May cause stomach upset.
Thiazides	Take with milk or food.

(Diuril, Hydrodiuril, other various brands)	Include high potassium foods in diet. Licorice may reduce the effect of these drugs.
Potassium Sparing **Spironolactone** (Aldactone)	May cause stomach upset. Take with milk or food.
Dyazide, Maxzide	May need to limit high-potassium foods. Check with your doctor.
GASTROINTESTINAL PREPARATIONS	
Diphenoxylate (Lomotil)	*Avoid alcohol or other depressants such as tranquilizers or sedatives.*
Metoclopramide (Reglan)	Take 1/2 hour before meals. May cause drowsiness. *Avoid alcoholic beverages.*
Cimetidine (Tagamet)	Take before meals. Stagger doses of antacids.
Famotidine (Pepcid)	Absorption unaffected by food.
Nizatidine (Axid)	
Ranitidine (Zantac)	
Pantoprazole (Protenox)	
Omeprazole (Prilosec)	Take before any meal.
Lansoprazole (Prevacid)	
Rabeprazole (Aciphex)	

Laxatives (Colace, Metamucil)	Take with 8 ounces of water.
MONOAMINE OXIDASE (MOA) INHIBITORS	**Patients on these medications should receive further instructions from their physician.**
Phenylzine (Nardil) **Tranylcypromine** (Parnate)	*Avoid foods high in tyramine while on these drugs (see Foods High in Tyramine chart). Avoid the herbal product St. John's Wort.*
MINERALS	
Iron (Fergon, Feosol, Ferrous sulfate, other various brands)	Take after meals or with food. *Do not take with tetracycline or antacids.*
Potassium Chloride (Micro-K, K-Dur)	May cause stomach upset. Take after meals or with food and a full glass of water.
HYPOGLYCEMIC AGENTS (Diabetes Medications)	
Insulin	Consult with your dietician or doctor about diet and exercise.
Chlorpropamide (Diabinese)	May cause stomach upset. Take with milk or food. *Avoid alcoholic beverages.*
Glipizide (Glucotrol)	Take 1/2 hour before meals.
Nateglinide (Starlix)	Take 1/2 hour before meals.
Glyburide (Diabeta, Micronase) **Metformin** (Glucophage) **Glimepiride** (Amaryl)	Take with meals.

Acarbose (Precose)	Take with the first bite of each meal.
Rosiglitazone (Avandia) **Pioglitizone** (Actos)	May take with or without meals.
MISCELLANEOUS	
Albuterol (Proventil, Ventolin)	May cause stomach upset. Take with milk or food.
Alendronate (Fosamax)	Take 1/2 hour before meals with a full glass of water.
Alprazolam (Xanax)	Take with milk or food. *Avoid alcoholic beverages.*
Antidepressants **Amitriptylline** (Elavil) **Citalopram** (Celexa) **Fluoxetine** (Prozac) **Paroxetine** Paxil **Sertraline** (Zoloft) **others**	*Avoid alcoholic beverages.* *Avoid the herbal product St. John's Wort.*
Antihistamines (Benadryl)	May cause stomach upset. Take with milk or food. Often causes drowsiness. *Avoid alcoholic beverages.*
Barbituates (Phenobarbital)	May cause drowsiness. *Do not take with alcoholic beverages or medicines with antihistamines. Avoid the following herbals: Wormwood, sage, evening primrose oil.*

Carbidopa/Levodopa (Sinemet)	May cause stomach upset. Take with food.
Corticosteroids **Prednisone** (Deltasone) **Prednisolone** (Delta-Cortef) **Hydrocortisone** (Deltef)	May cause stomach upset. Take with milk or food.
Lithium (Lithane, Eskalith)	May cause drowsiness. *Avoid alcoholic beverages.* Take after meals or with milk or food. Maintain consistent salt and fluid intake. Check with your doctor.
Meclizine (Antivert, Bonine)	May cause drowsiness. *Avoid alcoholic beverages.*
Phenytoin (Dilantin)	Take with food to increase absorption and reduce stomach irritation. *Avoid alcoholic beverages. Avoid the following herbal products: Wormwood, sage, GLA (evening primrose oil), shankapulshpi, epedra/Ma huang.*
Theophylline (TheoDur, Slo-bid, etc.)	May cause stomach upset. Take with food and water. Side effects are increased by caffeinated foods such as coffee, cocoa, cola, and chocolate. *Avoid the following herbal products: ephedra /Ma huang, guarana, kola, yohimbe.*

Food Information List

Note: *This list is not entirely inclusive. For more information, please consult with your dietitian or doctor.*

FOODS HIGH IN VITAMIN K

Asparagus	Cauliflower	Green beans	Soybean oil
Broccoli	Dark Lettuce	Green tea	Spinach
Cabbage	Garbanzo beans	Liver	Turnip greens

FOODS HIGH IN POTASSIUM

Fruits

Apricots (dried)	Dried fruit	Nectarines	Pomegranates
Bananas	Figs	Oranges (juice)	Prunes (juice)
Cantaloupe	Honeydew	Papaya	Raisins
Dates	Kiwi	Pears	

Vegetables

Artichokes	Beans (dried)	Peas	Sweet potatoes
Asparagus	Brussels sprouts	Potatoes	Tomatoes (juice)
Avocados	Carrots	Spinach (boiled)	Bamboo shoots
Parsnips	Squash		

FOODS HIGH IN TYRAMINE

Aged cheese	Broad beans	Pickled herring	Smoked fish
Aged meat	Caffeine *(limit)*	Raisins *(limit)*	Sour cream *(limit)*
Anchovies	Chocolate *(limit)*	Raspberries *(limit)*	Soy Sauce *(limit)*
Avocados *(limit)*	Canned figs *(limit)*	Sauerkraut	Yeast extract
Buttermilk *(limit)*	Liver	Sausages	Yogurt *(limit)*

Beverages High in Tyramine

Alcohol-free beer	Cola drinks
Beer and ale	Wine *(Chianti and Sherry)*

DRUGS AFFECTED BY GRAPEFRUIT JUICE*
Recent medical research has shown that grapefruit may interact with some drugs. For further information, please consult with your doctor and pharmacist.

*A residual effect may occur up to 24 hours or more after eating grapefruit or drinking grapefruit juice. This includes grapefruit supplements, grapefruit *in* supplements, grapefruit candies, and fruit drinks (including cocktails) made with grapefruit or grapefruit juice.

Consider avoiding grapefruit in any form while on the following medicines:

Alprazolam	Amlodipine	Atorvastatin	Buspirone
Caffeine	Carbamazepine	Caredilol	Clomipramine
Cyclosporine	Diazepam	Diltiazem	Dofetilide
Erythromycin	Estrogens	Felodipine	Fexofenadine
Itraconazole	Losartan	Lovastatin	Methylprednisone
Midazolam	Nicardipine	Nifedipine	Nisoldipine
Quinidine	Sawuinavir	Simvastatin	Tacrolimus
Terfenadine	Triazolam	Verapamil	

DRUGS AFFECTED BY HERBAL SUPPLEMENTS
Many herbal supplements and alternative medicines can interact with medicines you may already be taking or are starting to take. Inform your doctor and pharmacist if you are taking or plan to take any herbal, "natural," or "alternative" medicines, including any and all vitamin and/or mineral supplements, amino acids, or botanicals.

For more information contact:
Poudre Valley Hospital
Telephone: 970-495-7500
Public Relations: 970-237-7003
Website: www.pvhs.org

335

For additional information on various food, herb, alcohol,
and drug interactions visit:
http://www.fda.gov/consumer/updates/interactions112808.html

To visit the FDA's Drug Development and Drug Interactions website
go to:
www.fda.gov/cder/drug/drugInteractions/default.htm

To access Memorial Sloan-Kettering Cancer Center's database of
herbs, botanicals, and supplements go to:
http://www.mskcc.org/mskcc/html/11570.cfm

For further information on botanicals visit:
http://ods.od.nih.gov/factsheets/BotanicalBackground.asp

To download a sample medicine record go to:
www.fda.gov/cder/consumerinfo/my_medicine_record.htm

Appendix A

The following table devised by nutrition specialists at Virginia Tech offers an overview of safe storage durations for a variety of foods.

* Opened   ^ Refrigerate after opening
+ Cooked   # After manufacture date

Food	Pantry (Room Temperature)	Refrigerator (33°F to 40°F)	Freezer (0°F)
Bread and Cereal Products			
Baked quick breads	4-5 days	1-2 weeks	2-3 months
Bread	5-7 days	1-2 weeks	3 months
Bread crumbs and croutons	6 months		
Bread rolls, unbaked		2-3 weeks	1 month
Cereals, ready-to-eat	1 year 2-3 months*		
Cereals, ready-to-cook	6 months		
Corn meal	1 year	18 months	2 years
Doughnuts	4-5 days		3 months
Flour, cake, all-purpose	1 year		1-2 years
Flour, whole wheat		6-8 months	1-2 years
Pasta	2 years		
Pies and pastries		3 days	4-6 months
Pies and pastries, baked			1-2 months
Pies and pastries, cream filled		2-3 days	3 months
Pizza		3-4 days	1-2 months
Rice, brown	6 months		
Rice, white	1 year	6-7 days+	6 months+

Food	Pantry (Room Temperature)	Refrigerator (33°F to 40°F)	Freezer (0°F)
Tacos, enchiladas, and burritos (frozen)		2 weeks	1 year
Waffles		4-5 days	1 month
Packaged Foods and Mixes			
Biscuit, brownie, and muffin mixes	9 months		
Cakes, prepared	2-4 days		2-3 months
Cake mixes	6-9 months		
Casserole mix	9-12 months		
Chili powder	6 months		
Cookies, packaged	2 months		8-12 months
Crackers, pretzels	3 months		
Frosting, canned	3 months		
Frosting, mix	8 months		
Fruit cake		2-3 months	1 year
Hot roll mix	18 months		
Instant breakfast products	6 months		
Pancake and piecrust mix	6 months		
Pancake waffle batter		1-2 days	3 months
Toaster pastries	3 months		
Sauce and gravy mixes	6 months		
Soup mixes	1 year		
Spices, Herbs, Condiments, Extracts			
Catsup, chili, and cocktail sauce	1 year 1 month*	6 months	
Herbs	6 months		1-2 years
Herb/spice blends	2 years 1 year *		1-2 years

Food	Pantry (Room Temperature)	Refrigerator (33°F to 40°F)	Freezer (0°F)
Mustard	2 years	6-8 months*	8-12 months
Spices, ground	6 months		1-2 years
Spices, whole	1-2 years		2-3 years
Vanilla extract	2 years / 1 year*		
Other extracts	1 year		
Other Food Staples			
Bacon bits	4 months		
Baking powder	18 months		
Baking soda	2 years		
Bouillon products	1 year		
Carbonated soft drinks (12 oz. cans)	6-9 months		
Carbonated soft drinks, diet (12 oz. cans)	3-4 months		
Chocolate, premelted	1 year		
Chocolate syrup	2 years	6 months*	
Chocolate, semisweet	2 years		
Chocolate, unsweetened	18 months		
Cocoa mixes	8 months		
Coconut, shredded	1 year 6 months*	8 months	1 year
Coffee cans	2 years 2 weeks*	2 months	6 months
Coffee, instant	6 months 2 weeks*		
Coffee, vacuum-packed	1 year ^		
Coffee lighteners (dry)	9 months 6 months*		1 year

Food	Pantry (Room Temperature)	Refrigerator (33°F to 40°F)	Freezer (0°F)
Cornstarch	18 months		2 years
Gelatin	18 months		
Honey, jams, jellies, and syrup	1 year	6-8 months*	
Marshmallows	2-3 months		
Marshmallow cream	3-4 months		
Mayonnaise	2-3 months	12 months 2 months*	
Molasses	2 years		
Nuts, shelled	4 months	6 months	
Nuts, unshelled	6 months		
Nuts, salted			6-8 months
Nuts, unsalted			9-12 months
Oil, salad	3 months^ 2 months*		
Parmesan grated cheese	10 months 2 months*		
Pasteurized process cheese spread	3 months	3-4 weeks*	4 months
Peanut butter	6 months 2-3 months*		
Popcorn	1-2 years	2 years	2-3 years
Pectin	1 year		
Salad dressings, bottled	1 year^	3 months*	
Soft drinks	3 months		
Artificial sweetener	2 years		
Sugar, brown	4 months		
Sugar, confectioners	18 months		
Sugar, granulated	2 years		

Food	Pantry (Room Temperature)	Refrigerator (33°F to 40°F)	Freezer (0°F)
Tea bags	18 months		
Tea, instant	2 years		
Vegetable oils	6 months 1-3 months*		
Vegetable shortening	3 months	6-9 months	
Vinegar	2 years 1 year*		
Water, bottled	1-2 years		
Whipped topping (dry)	1 year		
Yeast, dry	Pkg. exp. date		
Vegetables			
Asparagus		2-3 days	8 months
Beets		2 weeks	
Broccoli		3-5 days	
Brussels sprouts		3-5 days	
Cabbage		1 week	
Carrots		2 weeks	
Cauliflower		1 week	
Celery		1 week	
Corn (husks)		1-2 days	8 months
Cucumbers		1 week	
Eggplant		1 week	
Green beans		1-2 days	8 months
Green peas		3-5 days	8 months
Lettuce		1 week	
Lima beans		3-5 days	8 months

341

Food	Pantry (Room Temperature)	Refrigerator (33°F to 40°F)	Freezer (0°F)
Mushrooms		2 days	
Onions	1 week	3-5 days	
Onion rings (precooked, frozen)			1 year#
Peppers		1 week	
Pickles, canned	1 year	1 month*	
Frozen potatoes			8 month
Sweet potatoes	2-3 weeks		
White potatoes	2-3 months		
Potato chips	1 month		
Radishes		2 weeks	
Rhubarb		3-5 days	
Rutabagas	1 week		
Snap beans		1 week	
Spinach		5-7 days	8 months
Squash, Summer		3-5 days	
Squash, Winter	1 week		
Tomatoes		1 week	
Turnips		2 weeks	
Commercial baby food, jars	1-2 years^	2-3 days	
Canned vegetables	1 year^	1-4 days*	
Canned vegetables, pickled	1 year^	1-2 months*	
Dried vegetables	6 months		
Frozen vegetables			8 months
Vegetable soup		3-4 days	3 months
Fruits			
Apples	Until ripe	1 month	

Food	Pantry (Room Temperature)	Refrigerator (33°F to 40°F)	Freezer (0°F)
Apricots	Until ripe	5 days	
Avocados	Until ripe	5 days	
Bananas	Until ripe	5 days (fully ripe)	
Berries	Until ripe	3 days	1 year
Canned fruit	1 year	2-4 days*	
Canned fruit juices	1 year	3-4 days*	
Cherries	Until ripe	3 days	
Citrus fruit	Until ripe	2 weeks	
Dried fruit	6 months	2-4 days+	
Frozen fruit			1 year
Fruit juice concentrate		6 days	1 year
Fruit pies, baked		2-3 days	8 months
Grapes	Until ripe	5 days	
Melons	Until ripe	5 days	
Nectarines	Until ripe	5 days	
Peaches	Until ripe	5 days	1 year
Pears	Until ripe	5 days	1 year
Pineapple	Until ripe	5-7 days	1 year
Plums	Until ripe	5 days	
Dairy Products			
Butter		1-2 months	9 months
Buttermilk		2 weeks	
Cottage cheese		1 week	3 months
Cream cheese		2 weeks	
Cream-light, heavy, half-and-half		3-4 days	1-4 months

Food	Pantry (Room Temperature)	Refrigerator (33°F to 40°F)	Freezer (0°F)
Eggnog (commercial)		3-5 days	6 months
Margarine		4-5 months	12 months
Condensed, evaporated & dry milk	12-23 months^	8-20 days*	
Milk		8-20 days	
Ice cream and sherbet			2 months
Hard natural cheese (e.g., cheddar, swiss)		3-6 months 4 weeks*	6 months
Hard natural cheese, sliced		2 weeks	
Processed cheese		1 month	6 months
Soft cheese (e.g., brie)		1 week	6 months
Pudding		1-2 days*	
Snack dips		1 week*	
Sour cream		2 weeks	
Non-dairy whipped cream, canned		3 months	
Real whipped cream, canned		3-4 weeks	
Yogurt		2 weeks	1-2 months
Meats, Poultry, Eggs, and Fish			
Meats			
Fresh beef and bison steaks		3-5 days	6-9 months
Fresh beef and bison roasts		3-5 days	9-12 months
Fresh pork chops		2-3 days	4-6 months
Fresh lamb chops		3-5 days	6-8 months
Fresh veal		1-2 days	4-6 months
Fresh ground meat (e.g. beef, lamb)		1 day	3-4 months
Cooked meat		2-3 days	2-3 months
Canned meat	1 year	3-4 days*	3-4 months

Food	Pantry (Room Temperature)	Refrigerator (33°F to 40°F)	Freezer (0°F)
Ham, whole		1 week	1-2 months
Ham, canned	1 year	1 week*	3-4 months
Ham, canned "keep refrigerated"		6-9 months 1 week*	3-4 months
Shelf-stable unopened canned meat (e.g. chili, deviled ham, corn beef)	1 year	1week*	
Ham, cook before eating		1 week	
Ham, fully cooked		2 weeks 1 week*	
Ham, dry-cured	1 year	1 month	
Ham salad, store prepared or homemade		3-5 days	
Bacon		2 weeks 1 week*	1 month
Corned beef, uncooked		5-7 days	1-2 months
Restructured (flaked) meat products			9-12 months
Sausage, fresh		1-2 days	1-2 months
Smoked breakfast sausage links, patties		1 week	2 months
Sausage, smoked (e.g., Mettwurst)		1 week	1-2 months
Sausage, semi-dry (e.g., Summer sausage)		2-3 weeks*	6 months
Sausage, dry smoked (e.g., Pepperoni, jerky, dry Salami)	1 year	1 month*	6 months
Frankfurters, bologna		2 weeks 3-5 days*	1-2 months
Luncheon meat		2 weeks 3-5 days*	1 month

Food	Pantry (Room Temperature)	Refrigerator (33°F to 40°F)	Freezer (0°F)
Meat gravies		1-2 days	2-3 months
TV beef and pork dinners			18 months#
Meat based casseroles		3-4 days	4 months
Variety meats (giblets, tongue, liver, heart, etc.)		1-2 days	3-4 months
Vinegar pickled meats (e.g. pickled pigs feet)	1 year^	2 weeks*	
Fish			
Breaded fish			4-6 months
Canned fish	1 year	1-2 days*	
Cooked fish or seafood		3-4 days	3 months
Lean fish (e.g. cod, flounder, haddock)		1-2 days	6 months
Fatty fish (e.g. bluefish, salmon, mackeral)		1-2 days	2-3 months
Dry pickled fish		3-4 weeks	
Smoked fish		2 weeks	4-5 weeks
Seafood-clams, crab, lobster in shell		2 days	3 months
Seafood-oysters and scallops		1-2 days	3-4 months
Seafood-shrimp		1-2 days	1 year
Seafood-shucked clams		1-2 days	3-6 months
Tuna salad, store prepared or homemade		3-5 days	
Poultry and Eggs			
Chicken nuggets or patties		1-2 days	
Chicken livers		1-2 days	3 months
Chicken and poultry TV dinners			6 months

Food	Pantry (Room Temperature)	Refrigerator (33°F to 40°F)	Freezer (0°F)
Canned poultry^	1 year	1 day*	
Cooked poultry		2-3 days	4-6 months
Fresh poultry		1 day	1 year
Frozen poultry parts			6-9 months
Canned poultry		1 day	3 months
Poultry pies, stews, and gravies		1-2 days	6 months
Poultry salads, store prepared or homemade		3-5 days	
Poultry stuffing, cooked		3-4 days	1 month
Eggs, in shell		3-5 weeks	
Eggs, hard-boiled		1 week	
Eggs, pasteurized		10 days 3 days*	1 year
Egg substitute		10 days 3 days*	1 year
Egg yolks (covered in water)		2-4 days	1 year
Egg whites (For each cup of egg yolk add 1 Tbs. of sugar or salt)		2-4 days	1 year
Wild Game			
Frog legs		1 day	6-9 months
Game birds		2 days	9 months
Small game (rabbit, squirrel, etc.)		2 days	9-12 months
Venison ground meat		1-2 days	2-3 months
Venison steaks and roasts		3-5 days	9-12 months

Table provided by Virginia Tech:
http://www.ext.vt.edu/pubs/foods/348-960/348-960.html

Index

C

Caffeine, 24, 47
  and potential health problems, 96
  danger to animals, 96
  drug interactions with, 100-101
  drug interactions with, 98-99
  in chocolate, 95, 96
Calcium, 182-184
  absorption of, 182-183
  and alcohol intake, 183
  and lactose, 182
  and oxalates, 182-183
  fiber and, 182-183
  in canned bony fish, 92
  tannins and, 182-183
Calories
  from fat, 273-274
Campylobacter jejuni, 205-206, 220, 237
Cancer, 298-299
  and heterocyclic amines, 298
  and obesity, 307
  overcooked pork as risk factor, 91
Candidiasis, 321
Cane sugar
  chemical residues in, 113
  cons of, 113
  pros of, 113
CAP-RAST, 319
Carbohydrates, 131-135
  and alcohol, 134-135
  and dieting, 133-135
  and ketosis, 134
  complex, 133
  simple, 132
  types of, 131-133
Carbon monoxide
  and beef, 90
Carbon, 137-141
Carmine, 286
Carotid artery disease, 300
Carrageenan, 52

CDC, 81, 223, 229, 231, 232, 306
Celiac disease, 313-314
  and type 1 diabetes, 313
  bread consumption and, 88
  oats and, 104
  rice and, 103
Center for Food Safety, 84
Center For Science in the Public Interest, 84, 157
Cephalosporins, 220
Cereal
  cons of, 116-117
  pros of, 116
Cheese
  per capita consumption of, 38
Chefs
  as source of nutritional information, 31
Chemical residues
  in soy, 106
Chemical toxins, 218
Chemicals, 235
  food development and, 226-227
Chemotherapy
  and effects on nutrition, 58
  food preparation and, 43
Chicken
  and foodborne illness, 94
  cons of, 94
  pros of, 93-94
Children
  and lead ingestion, 321
  nutritional needs of, 260-261
Chloride, 185
Chocolate, 14, 94-96
  acne and, 94
  and cough suppression, 95
  antioxidants in, 94
  caffeine in, 95, 96
  cons of, 96
  pros of, 94-95
  theobromine in, 95, 96
Choice-related variables, 18-20

351

natural sugar content of, 51
pasteurization of, 50
preservatives in, 50
types of, 50-51

K

Kidney disease, 302

L

Labeling (see also *food labeling*)
allergies and, 235
error-related variables and, 21
exemption from, 23
organics, 248, 249-250
organics, 250
requirements, 23
Labels
nutritional information on, 31
Lactase enzyme, 39
Lactase, 151
Lactitol, 155
Lactobacillus acidophilus, 108
Lactobacillus bifidus, 108
Lactobacillus, 201
Lactose intolerance, 39, 152
Lactose, 38, 39, 132, 151
Laxatives, 309
LDL cholesterol, 138, 140, 143
Lead, 56
in ceramic cookware, 56
ingestion by children, 321
Levulose, 132, 149
Lind, James, 159
Linoleic acid, 138
Linseed, 139
Lipase, 198
Lipids, 137
Liquid sugar, 151-152
Listeria monocytogenes, 21, 208-210
Listeriosis, 209
and meningitis, 209
and pregnancy complications, 209, 210

and septicemia, 209
Lithium, and abrupt caffeine withdrawal, 99, 101
Liver disease, 305
Livestock
and error-related variables, 20-21
Low-density lipoprotein (LDL), 138, 296, 297, 298
Lutein, 101
in eggs, 107
Lycopene, tomatoes, 41
Lysine
herpes simplex and, 108
in dairy products, 108

M

Macrominerals, 182-188
Mad cow disease, 21, 218, 239
scrapie-infected sheep and, 21
Magnesium, 186-187
Maine lobsters
and risk of Paralytic Shellfish Poisoning, 93
Maize, 150
Males
nutritional needs of, 264
Malt extract, 152
Malt sugar, 152
Malt syrup, 152
Maltitol, 155
Maltodextrin, 148, 152
Maltose, 132, 152
Manganese, 193
Mannitol, 155
Maple syrup, 152-153
Margarine, 15
Marketing, 78
cons of, 64-65
pros of, 64
Meat, 33
antibiotics in, 34
color enhancers in, 34
cut and grade of, 33

bleached, 102
bromated, 102
chemical residues in, 102
cons of, 102
pros of, 101
Whiskey
production of, 50
WIC, 77
Willet, Walter C., 123, 124
Wine, 49, 82
labeling of, 72
lead content in, 115
manufacture of, 49
regulation of, 82
resveratrol, 115
safety of, 72
sulfites in, 49
Winter, Ruth, 293
World Food Safety Organization, 83
World Health Organization, 45, 83
Wort syrup, 155

X

Xylitol, 155

Y

Yeast infection, 321
Yersinia enterocolitica, 210-211

Z

Zeaxanthin, 101
in eggs, 107
Zinc, 190-192
Zoochemicals, 198-199

Notes

Notes

Notes

Notes

Order Form

Copies of *FoodSmart* are $21.95 plus shipping. Florida residents please add 6% sales tax. Checks and money orders (U.S. funds) accepted. **MasterCard and Visa orders only call 800.266.5752.**

Name_____

Address_____

City_____State_____ Zip_____

Phone_____Email_____

    ____ copies @ $21.95 =   _____
6% sales tax (FL residents only)   _____1.31_____
Shipping/Handling
($5.95 Book Rate; $7.95 Priority
Mail per copy)   _____

TOTAL   _____

Mail your order to:

**Consumer Press
Order Department FS1
13326 Southwest 28th Street, Suite 102
Fort Lauderdale, FL 33330-1102**

**Credit Card Orders: 800.266.5752 / 954.370.9153
Online Orders: www.consumerpress.com**